Praise for *Honey, Have You Squeezed the Dachshund*

"*Honey, Have You Squeezed the Dachshund?* is a must-have for dachshund owners! Even if you are not currently dealing with IVDD, the information is invaluable. When I adopted my first IVDD dog over 10 years ago, I had to learn how to care for him all on my own. A book like this would have saved me lots of headaches, and lots of carpet cleaning! The authors have brought it all together in a simple, concise, and humorous way to let dachshund parents know what to expect before, during, and after an IVDD episode. The charts and checklists will help you navigate the 'what ifs' of IVDD. From having proactive conversations with your veterinarian, to crate rest, treatment and therapy options, to daily care of an IVDD dog (including the squeezing of the bladder!), this is a book you need!"

—Angela Johnston, dachshund mom to Skippy (IVDD survivor and multiple champion of the National Dachshund Races wheelchair division) and Maggie (IVDD survivor)

"Brilliant. Makes a complicated disease and situation easy to understand from not only the medical aspect but the emotional stress and heartbreak that pet owners feel. Extremely informative and emotionally supportive. I will be buying copies to give to all of my clients when they bring their dogs in to my office for this disease. Thank you for writing such a great resource for my clients and patients!"

—Dr. Annie Price, DVM, Atlanta, Georgia

"Every dachshund should come with this book attached to the collar! While we all hope our dog is never diagnosed with IVDD, education is key. Kristin Leydig Bryant and Dr. Adam Christman have done a valuable service in putting together this very detailed book on how to live with, and care for, a dog with IVDD; how to be prepared ahead of time should this happen to your pup; and how a dog with IVDD can thrive! The added touch of humor in this book, I can personally attest, is the medicine that got me through when my dachshund became paralyzed. The best thing you'll get from this book? Hope! There is always hope!"

—Barbara Techel, founder of The Frankie Wheelchair Fund and National Walk 'N Roll Dog Day, author of *Through Frankie's Eyes: One Woman's Journey to Her Authentic Self, and the Dog on Wheels Who Led the Way*, plus two children's books about her paralyzed dachshund, Frankie (the Walk 'N Roll Dog)

"In *Honey, Have You Squeezed the Dachshund?* you will find the gift of knowledge and strength to help you help your longdog. Read it. Highlight important sections. If you have a dachshund (or any longbodied dog) of any age, this book will guide you through coping with IVDD, whether your dog is in an active episode or in recovery. IVDD dogs know joy, love, and doxietude! IVDD dogs are tenacious, strong, and whether they have wheels or four paws on the floor, they are ready for action!"

—Brenda Johnson, co-founder of K9BackPack.com and Getalongdog Rescue; dachshund mom to Billie (IVDD survivor) and Freddie

"Will make even the most insecure person feel as though they can tackle anything that comes their way if their dog should go down with IVDD."

—Carole Harden Taylor, rescue advocate and admin for Celebrating Dachshunds Facebook Group; dachshund mom to Ruby, Wolfgang (IVDD survivor), Marlee, and Stanley

"I have been a mom to IVDD and paralyzed dogs for many years and have managed countless IVDD patients in practice—this information is spot-on! A fantastic, well-written, informative, easy to understand, and entertaining guidebook on how to manage your dog's health and well-being if he or she develops a back problem or becomes paralyzed. This book addresses not only what to do and what not to do, but additionally touches on the difficult emotions we often have surrounding the diagnosis, treatment, choices, and management of our fur-children in these stressful circumstances. Everyone with a dachshund or long-back dog should read this—I will undoubtedly be recommending this book to all of my long-back dog owners."

—Dr. Carolyn Karrh, DVM, Denver, Colorado

"This book lets you know that you and your ween are NOT alone. There are things you can do starting right away to make a bad situation not so bad, and even make it better."

—Regina Reif, RVT and dachshund mom to Zooey and Paddington

Honey, Have You Squeezed the Dachshund?

A Guide for Dachshund Owners Who Are Terrified of IVDD

By Kristin Leydig Bryant and Adam Christman, DVM, MBA
With illustrations by Kelly Guntner

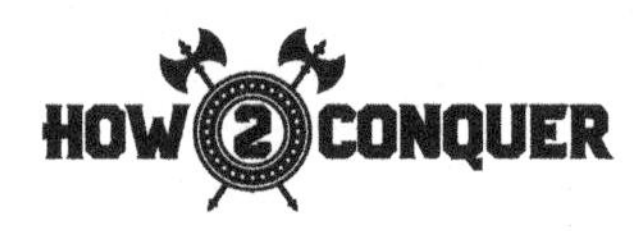

Published by How2Conquer
1298 Metropolitan Avenue SE
Atlanta, Georgia 30316
www.how2conquer.com

First edition, September 2016

Book cover and interior design by Kelly Guntner
Edited by Grace Duggan
Kristin Leydig Bryant photograph by Rachel Iliadis
Adam Christman photograph by Christopher Zisko

Printed in the United States of America

ISBN 978-1-945783-00-5

dedication

for all the dogs whose lives we hope will be saved with this knowledge

"I think dogs are the most amazing creatures; they give unconditional love. For me they are the role model for being alive."

—Gilda Radner

table of contents

who are you? 1
help! my dachshund's back is hurt! the first 48 hours of IVDD 3
your veterinarian says it's IVDD. you're overwhelmed. 4
is IVDD really an injury, or is it a disease? 6
how bad could bad be? life with a down dachshund 8
ease up on the hair trigger, tex 10
the two basic treatment paths: surgery and crate rest 12
six things to consider when choosing your base treatment 13
what to expect with surgery 15
what to expect with crate rest 16
some final thoughts on choosing a treatment 18
part one: i think my dog has had an IVDD injury. what should i do? 21
the vet exam: what can i expect? 25
the neurological exam 27
know your Cs, Ts, and Ls 29
how do you decide? 30
part two: base treatment details 31
what to expect with IVDD surgery 31

the phone call ... 33
what to expect with crate rest ... 41
i can't do surgery or crate rest. i just can't. ... 57
part three: we got through the base treatment! what now? ... 63
the crazy ways function comes back ... 66
do we need more rehab? ... 68
part four: the paraplegic dachshund user manual ... 71
joining the bladder club (aka finding the bladder) ... 73
the urinary tract: what you need to know ... 75
a daily schedule ... 77
squeezing a girl ... 81
squeezing a boy ... 83
risks—guess what? bladder rupture isn't one of them ... 88
leaks are your fault, but you're still a good person ... 89
urinary tract infections in paraplegic dogs ... 90
the golden fluid: earning your pee-h-d ... 92
poops you can be proud of ... 93
the down-dog-friendly home and yard ... 99
skin concerns ... 100
part five: rollin', rollin', rollin'—wheelchair carts ... 105
when is it time to get a cart? ... 107
choosing a cart ... 108

used carts and DIY carts....112
the cart has arrived! now what do i do? 112
wheelchair fun....115
sling, batter batter! an alternative to wheelchair carts....116
preparation tools, glossary, and other resources....119
preparation tools: minimizing your risk and being prepared....120
glossary: the language of IVDD....128
resources....132
closing thoughts....135
will IVDD be around forever?....135
IVDD and further advances in treatment....137
you're an ambassador now 138
dogs and people to thank....139
about the authors and illustrator....141
sources consulted....144

who are you?

If you've picked up this book, you're probably one of three kinds of people.

1. Your dog has Intervertebral Disc Disease (IVDD), right now, and you're freaking out.

More than likely, the way you discovered IVDD was because your dachshund, or corgi, or basset hound, or other horizontally oriented dog was screaming in agony and shaking like a birch leaf. Perhaps she couldn't move her back legs and was dragging herself across the floor. You're probably feeling a terrible combination of fear, pity, panic, and helplessness. At the same time, you're picturing your last ATM balance and wondering whether you can afford any of this, and whether you can live with yourself if you can't afford it—whatever "it" is.

So you looked up IVDD online, or maybe your veterinarian handed this book to you, and here we are.

You'll want to start with "Help, My Dachshund's Back Is Hurt! The First 48 Hours" on page 3 and read straight through. Later, when you have more time to breathe, you can get more details in the rest of the book.

2. Your dog was diagnosed with IVDD a while ago, and you're ready for some tips and tricks.

You're through the horrific pain part, and now you want to figure out how to move forward. Maybe your dog is paralyzed, maybe she isn't, but you want to make sure you're doing everything you can to make her life happy. Start with "Part Four: The Paraplegic Dachshund User Manual" on page 71.

3. You're the proactive, self-educating type.

Good for you! You love one of those breeds that are prone to back issues, and you're trying to prepare yourself for what might happen. (By the way, we love you.) Read at your leisure.

If you're one of these three kinds of people, this book is for you!

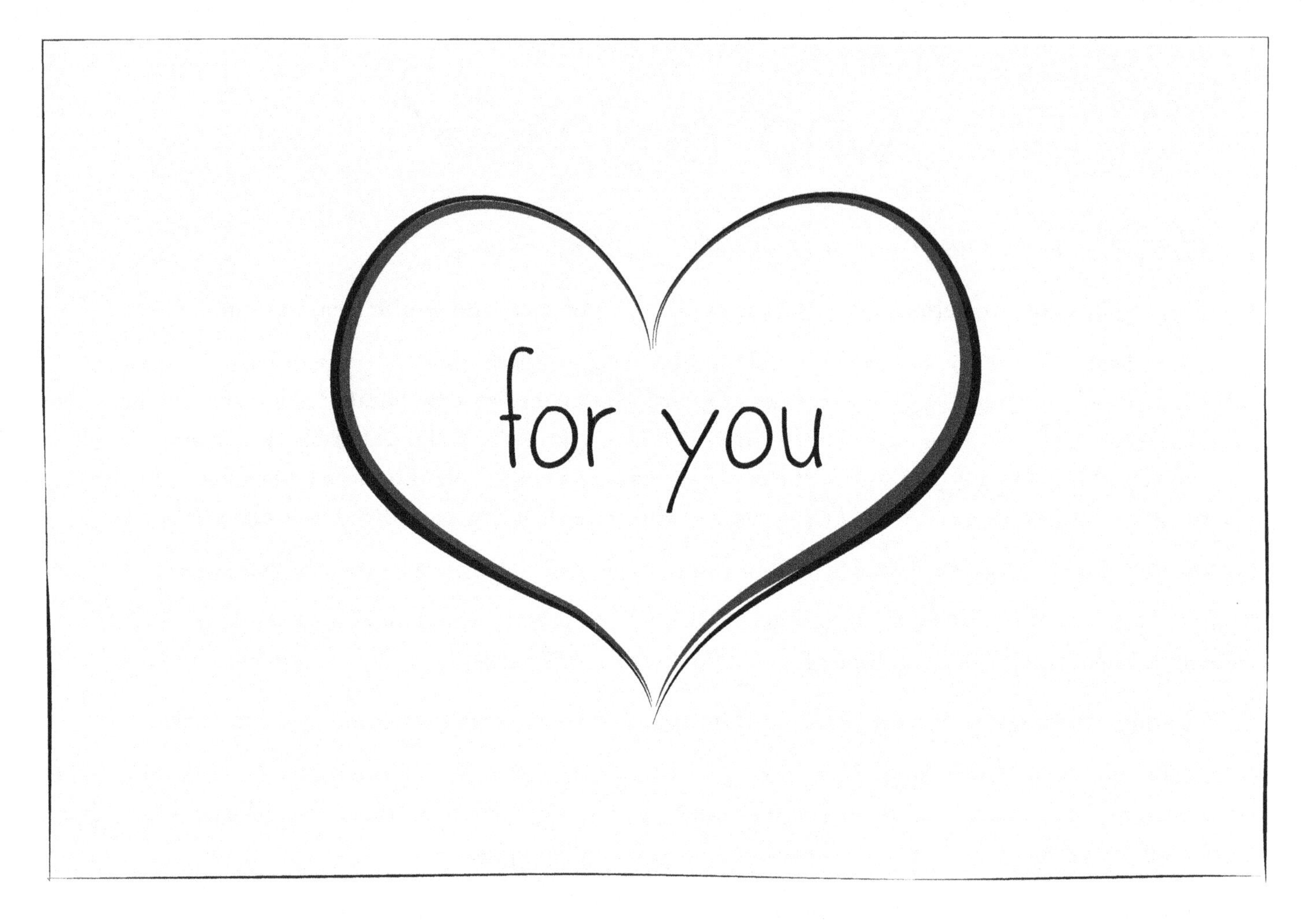

IVDD is terrible—there is no denying that. We are not making light of it, but we do try to use a little humor to get us through. Then again, maybe IVDD isn't *quite* as terrible as you think. (Once you get your dog past the screaming and trembling part, of course.) Maybe. With IVDD, there are no guarantees, and there are lots of variables.

In most situations, IVDD is not a death sentence. The scientific veterinary community is working on cool stuff like stem cell therapies and genetic modifications, and of course you'll want to know about all of that. At some point. But that's not what this book is for. This book will help you deal with some practicalities you can use in the short term. You're not alone. Lots of people have been there and gotten through it. You will too.

help! my dachshund's back is hurt! the first 48 hours of IVDD

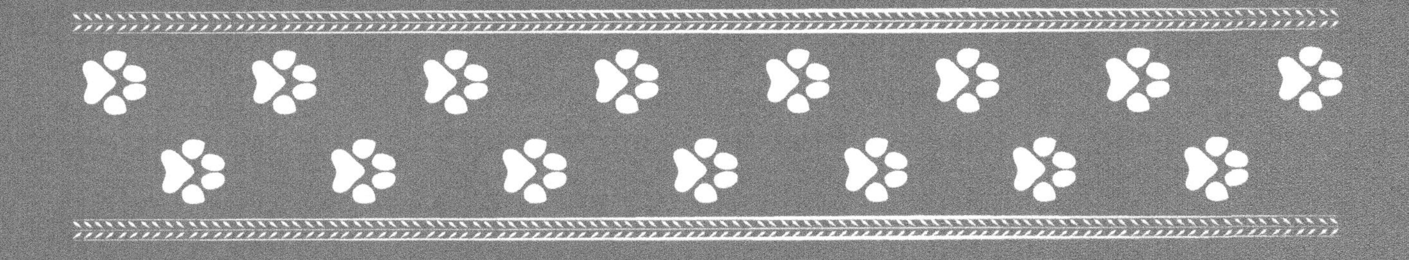

This section will help you get through the first 48 hours of an IVDD (intervertebral disc disease) flare-up. It's a summary of everything you absolutely need to know to wrap your mind around what is happening to your dog's back. You can find more detailed information further in the book.

your veterinarian says it's IVDD. you're overwhelmed.

Let's get some basic information into you. Just the facts for now.

- IVDD is an inherited condition, not an injury. It causes the discs in a dog's spine, which sit between each vertebra, to dry out and weaken. The weakened discs can swell or rupture, causing injury to the spinal cord. We call this a flare-up.
- The most common signs of an IVDD flare-up include crying, shaking, tight tummy, hunched back, and refusal to do things she normally does easily, like climb up one step. These are all signs of pain, and an IVDD flare-up usually causes a lot of pain.
- In some dogs, pain is the only symptom. Some dogs will also be paralyzed, usually in the rear legs. These dogs will either refuse to move at all, or they will drag themselves across the floor—a horrifying sight for the uninitiated. Some dogs will be paralyzed but not have pain. Some will also lose the ability to pee or poop independently.

IVDD is not...

- a broken back
- an old dog disease
- contagious
- breed-specific
- something you can just ignore and hope will go away

Most importantly, IVDD is not a death sentence.

- There are two basic treatment paths: 1) surgery and 2) strict crate rest with medications. Surgery removes the ruptured disc material that is pressing on the spinal cord and damaging it. Crate rest requires medication to reduce spinal cord swelling, and it depends on the body's ability to reabsorb the disc material before the spinal cord is permanently damaged. Your choice will depend on many factors.
- For surgery, you need a specialist. The most common procedure is called a hemilaminectomy. A regular veterinarian is not equipped to perform this procedure. The surgeon will relieve the pressure on the spinal cord by cleaning away the material that ruptured out of the disc. Surgery might also mean cutting an opening into the bone to give the swollen spinal cord some room.
- Some veterinarians do not recommend surgery unless the dog has lost the ability to walk.
- Surgery costs vary greatly from surgeon to surgeon. If possible, get an estimate from the surgeon directly. See page 14 for guidance.

- For strict crate rest with medications, you will keep your dog very still in a crate for eight weeks so that the swelling can subside and the spinal cord and disc(s) can heal. Drugs (commonly an anti-inflammatory, muscle relaxers, and others) are required to reduce swelling, control pain, and minimize muscle spasms.
- Neither surgery nor strict crate rest with medications is guaranteed to restore the ability to walk if a dog is paralyzed. Either will relieve pain in the majority of dogs. The more quickly you begin either treatment path, the better the chance of restoring function, i.e., the ability to walk and control the bladder again. (Throughout this book, when we refer to the bladder, we mean the urinary bladder, not the gall bladder.)
- Your dog may not walk again, whichever treatment path you choose. A paralyzed dachshund can have a happy life with minimal additional care. Yes, the care is different, but it is not much more trouble than taking care of an able-bodied dog. Quality of life can be just as high. Paralyzed dogs play, wrestle, chase toys, and even get into trouble, just like any other dog.
- You cannot do nothing. You have to do something. If your dog is in pain, doing nothing is not an act of love. You must relieve the pain.
- You cannot just give pain medications. Your dog needs the restriction of activity that crate rest ensures. Without crate rest, your dog will make the injury worse by jostling the spinal cord.
- Other therapies exist. Some common ones are laser, acupuncture, chiropractic, physical therapy, swim therapy, and various supplements and injections. Our experience has been that these therapies are not useful unless you also do either surgery or crate rest. Some can even be harmful at this stage.
- Many veterinarians recommend euthanasia for dachshunds who go "down" with IVDD, especially to clients who cannot afford surgery. At the "emergency" point in your process, we believe euthanasia is needed only when ALL of the following are true:

    1. You cannot provide surgery.
    2. You cannot spend eight weeks trying crate rest with meds.
    3. You cannot care for a disabled dog if treatment doesn't work.
    4. Your breeder will not accept the dog back within the next 24 hours.
    5. You cannot find a dachshund rescue or another qualified home to take her into their care within 24 hours.

is IVDD really an injury, or is it a disease?

disease
+ event
injury

IVDD is a disease, but you probably won't know your dog has it until it results in an injury. The disease of the disc can cause injury to the spinal cord, usually after an event like jumping off the sofa.

Picture your dog's spine as a long row of rings, like a kid's ring-toss game. Those are the vertebrae, made of hard bone. A cable runs through the holes. That cable is the spinal cord, your dog's information superhighway. Below the spinal cord, a row of little pillows keeps the hard rings from rubbing together. Those pillows are the discs.

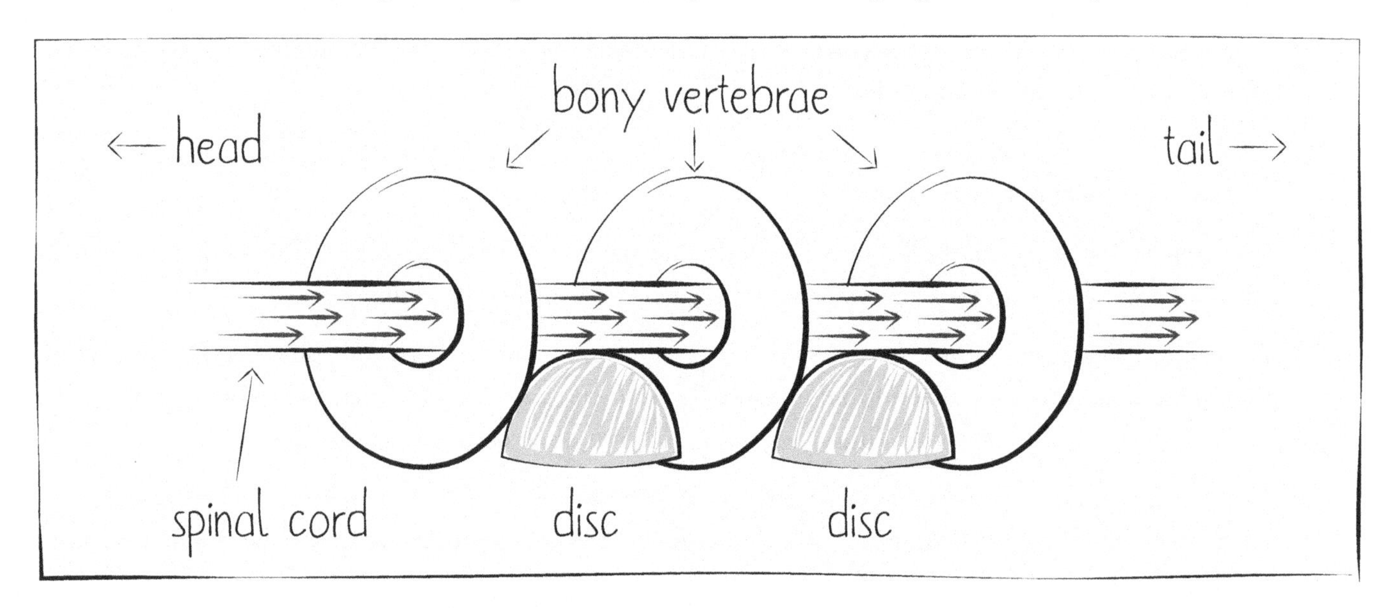

Why Is It Called IVDD?

Inter means between. The discs are little pillows that sit between the vertebrae.

Vertebral, of course, refers to the bones in the spine. The vertebrae get smaller and smaller as they go toward the tail. The spinal cord runs through the holes in the rings to carry all kinds of information from the brain to the rest of the body.

A **Disc** sits between the bottom half of each of the bony rings. Discs are made of a fibrous coating holding in a jelly-like center. (Picture a pillow made like a jelly doughnut.) The discs act as shock absorbers, keeping the vertebrae from grinding together. They also help the spine bend.

The **Disease** is the weakening of the discs. As the discs degenerate, the fibrous coating (the pillowcase) becomes dry and brittle, losing the ability to flex. This gradual hardening is called calcification. As a disc calcifies, it is more likely to allow the jelly-like part to swell or squirt out and wreak havoc on the sensitive spinal cord. Some veterinarians use the word Degeneration for the second D.

What Actually Happens?

If your dog was born with IVDD, the disease, the coating on her discs has become more dry and brittle with every year, and less able to hold the insulating jelly in.

If the jelly inside the disc bulges (or bursts out), it presses the cord up against the hard inside of the bony vertebra. If your dog is having trouble walking, the pressure is not only causing pain, it is also keeping signals from the brain from getting through to the rest of the body. It's like a garden hose that got pinched.

Most of the time, the flare-up (bulge or rupture) is caused by an event that pushes the jelly out of the disc through the brittle weak spot. Impacts are the most common events—jumping off something or running down stairs. This is most likely to happen between four and eight years of age. The most common age for the first event is five.

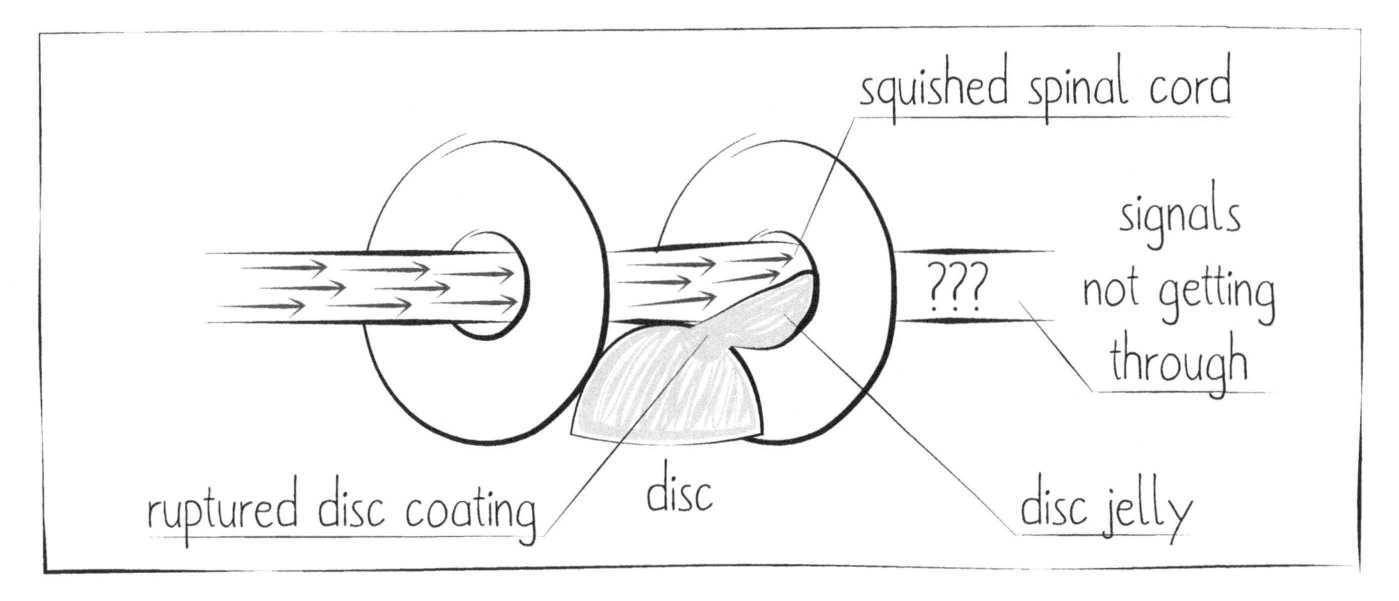

Remember—your dog already had IVDD. You just didn't know it until an event actually caused the jelly in the disc to injure the spinal cord.

What makes this especially frustrating is that unlike many other inherited diseases, IVDD cannot be identified at birth. But if breeders are keeping good records of their puppies' health after purchase, a good breeder would stop breeding the parents of dogs who turned out to have IVDD.

how bad could bad be? life with a down dachshund

The Down and the Dirty

You're probably wondering, especially if your vet doesn't sound too optimistic, *What if treatment doesn't work? If my dog were paraplegic, what would I need to do to take care of her? What would her life be like? What's all this bladder business about anyway?*

You have decisions to make. These are the things you need to know in the ultra-short term to understand what caring for a down dachshund is like—and that it doesn't have to be a Herculean task.

The four big concerns people have with these little guys are peeing, pooping, mobility, and attitude.

1. Peeing

- A down dachshund is not incontinent. She is the opposite of incontinent: She cannot urinate without help.
- Many down dachshunds need their bladders to be expressed (squeezed) for them.
- Squeezing a bladder is not difficult to learn. It takes about 20 seconds and requires no equipment besides your hands. You will not get pee on you while you do it. You can even do it over the toilet.
- A down dog needs to be squeezed about the same number of times a day as a normal dog goes outside to potty. You just keep them on a schedule. You can do it with a normal full time job.
- Pee will leak out only if the bladder is full to overflowing. Most down dachshunds do not need diapers.
- Down dachshunds can be prone to urinary tract infections (UTIs), but most of these are easily treated with antibiotics.

2. **Pooping**
    - Unlike peeing, a down dachshund does not need help pooping. Poop will come out on its own.
    - True, the poop will not always make its appearance at the most convenient time. You can learn to express the poop just as you do the pee. This is also easy. No, it does not involve rubber gloves or touching poop.
3. **Mobility**
    - Wheelchair carts, available online, come in several types and price points. Most dogs enjoy having a cart, especially for neighborhood walks.
    - Many people, including Dr. Christman, use a homemade sling made from a resistance band to take their dachshunds on walks.
    - Neither a cart nor a resistance band is necessary for just hanging around the house. Down dogs can shimmy around the house surprisingly quickly.
4. **Attitude**
    - Attitude is almost never an issue. These are dachshunds, after all. Badger dogs! Down dachshunds don't worry about the future. They don't look at other dogs, sigh wistfully, and remember when they too could run across the yard after that squirrel. No, down dachshunds just pull themselves recklessly at full speed across the yard after the squirrel.
    - Down dogs play, snuggle, beg, nap, wrestle, chase balls, and de-squeak stuffie toys. None of that changes just because their back legs don't work. As far as they are concerned, they are still dogs.
    - Paralyzed dogs do need more ear scratches, because they can't scratch their own ears. You're willing to do that, aren't you?

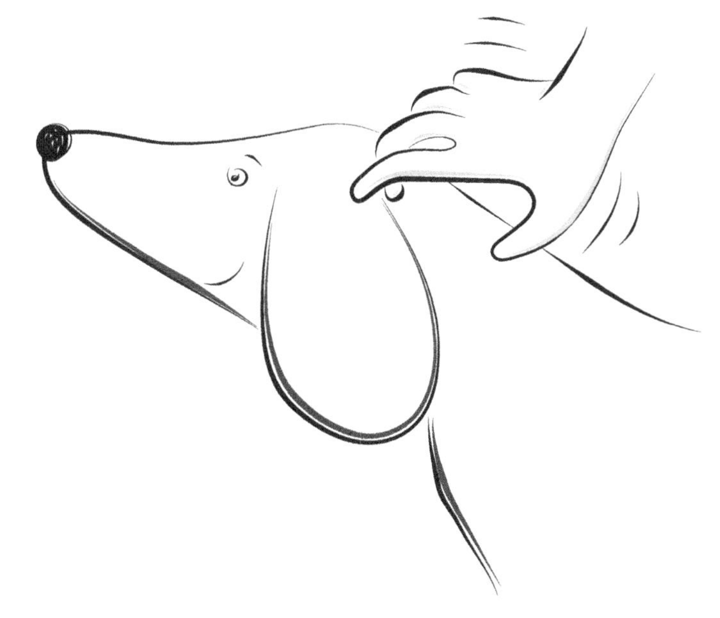

Really, caring for a down dachshund is not hard. It's different than caring for a dog with normal needs, but it isn't harder. But don't just take our word for it. You can see lots and lots of down dogs in action on the internet. Search for videos using any combination of these terms:

- Paralyzed + video + dachshund
- Paraplegic + video + dachshund
- IVDD + video + dachshund
- Wheelchair + video + dachshund (and, while you're at it, + race!)

Any of these will turn up videos of dachshunds doing what dachshunds do, who happen to also be paralyzed.

ease up on the hair trigger, tex

Don't Do Anything You Might Regret in 24 Hours

Let's deal with where you probably are as you read this. You're in the vet's office, maybe crying. The vet says that your dachshund will be paralyzed if she doesn't get surgery. She may be paralyzed even if she *does* get surgery. "What does that mean?" you ask. And the vet says, "She won't be able to walk, and she'll be incontinent, and you will have to express her bladder… every day."

Immediately, you picture your dog piteously dragging her half-useless, abraded body around the yard where she used to joyfully romp after butterflies. And this bladder expression business? You picture rubber hoses, latex gloves, kneeling by the bathtub with your bad knees, and a big, smelly mess several times a day. Maybe even catheters! (Although you are not quite sure what catheters are.) You imagine yourself up close and personal with dog urine. And worse.

You may be thinking, "I can't do that. I have a job! And a sensitive constitution!" Or, "She wouldn't want me to do that. She's an independent dog with a profound dignity of spirit."

Let's Talk Vocabulary for Just a Second

The word *express* is not a word we often encounter in this context, is it? To *express* the bladder just means to *empty* it—squeeze it until it empties. That's it! No equipment. Just your hands, which stay on the outside and don't touch the urine. You don't need to learn how to insert anything, or *where* to insert it. There is no inserting!

We like the word *express* because it implies *fast*, and expressing a bladder definitely is. It's quick, like an express train. Less than one minute. It's a lot quicker than waiting for your other dog to pee outside, when you're trying to get to work by 8 a.m., and she's moseying around exploring every random smell she somehow didn't get to the night before.

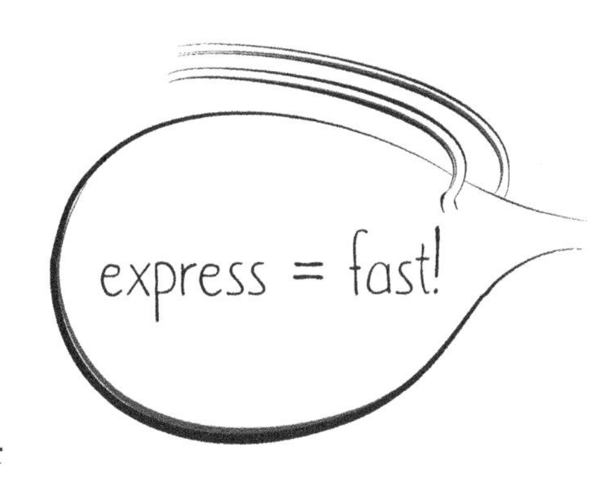

Secondly, the word *incontinent* isn't right. An incontinent dog can't hold her urine in. A paraplegic dog can't get her urine out without help. Big difference. So if you were imagining rivers of urine flowing behind your little dog everywhere she goes, please let that image go.

For Now, Buy Some Time

This is an emotional time of complicated decisions about things that are new. Your dog is trembling and wailing, and you've driven to a medical professional with your hands shaking on the steering wheel. You're distraught and panicked.

Right now, get your dog some pain relief. Once you have an IVDD diagnosis, that's Job #1. Your dog needs something strong to reduce the swelling and take some pressure off the spinal cord. Demand this as though you were Shirley MacLaine in *Terms of Endearment*. If you don't know this reference, stop reading and search for it online it so you have a useful model for the level of intensity you should employ in your request.

After the meds are on board, you will have a little bit of time to learn about the treatment paths, likelihood of recovery, worst-case scenarios, the dirty work, and whether you can handle it. You'll have some time to research a little bit, and to talk things over with your cabinet—your most trusted advisors, your besties, your family, and maybe the person who does your taxes.

Mind you, nothing has been fixed with the medications. You've just bought yourself a thinking period—24 hours, no more—so you can make good decisions calmly. While you figure everything out over the next day or so, your dog needs to be kept as still as possible in a crate, 24/7, whether that's at your house or at the vet, well-medicated.

There Is Hope

Maybe IVDD isn't quite as terrible as you think. (Once you get your dog past the screaming-in-agony part, of course.) There are different treatment options, but there are no guarantees, and there are lots of variables. In most situations, though, there is no reason for IVDD to be a death sentence.

the two basic treatment paths: surgery and crate rest

If you were at the IVDD Café—not a restaurant anyone would choose, of course—surgery or crate rest would be your two main dish choices, and other therapies would be available as side dishes or desserts.

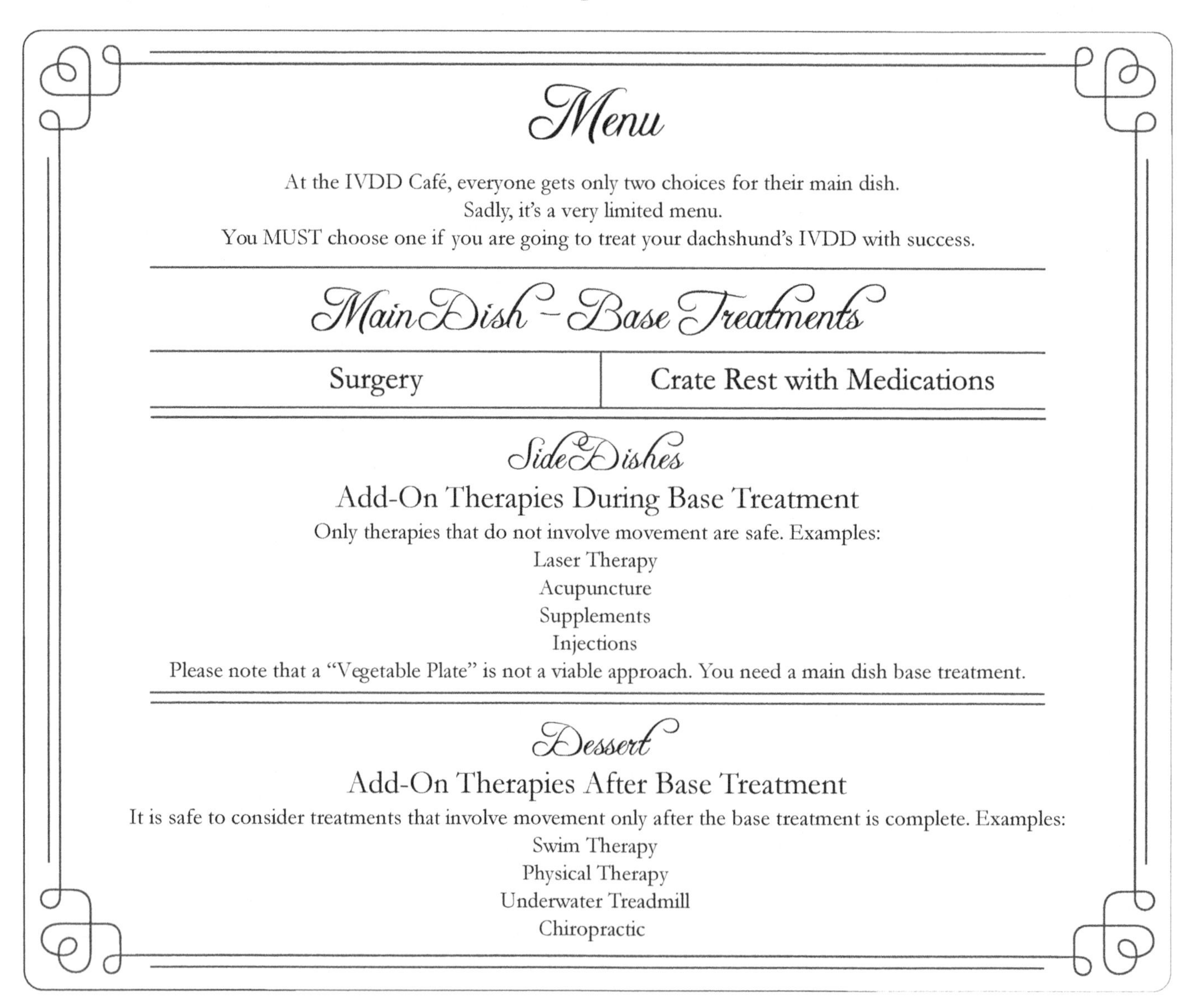

Menu

At the IVDD Café, everyone gets only two choices for their main dish.
Sadly, it's a very limited menu.
You MUST choose one if you are going to treat your dachshund's IVDD with success.

Main Dish - Base Treatments

Surgery	Crate Rest with Medications

Side Dishes

Add-On Therapies During Base Treatment

Only therapies that do not involve movement are safe. Examples:

Laser Therapy
Acupuncture
Supplements
Injections

Please note that a "Vegetable Plate" is not a viable approach. You need a main dish base treatment.

Dessert

Add-On Therapies After Base Treatment

It is safe to consider treatments that involve movement only after the base treatment is complete. Examples:

Swim Therapy
Physical Therapy
Underwater Treadmill
Chiropractic

six things to consider when choosing your base treatment

IVDD, like anything involving the nerves and brain signals, is a strange disease. It can be unpredictable. A lot of things can change the treatment outcome, whether you choose surgery or crate rest. It's complicated.

Time

How much time passed before you recognized symptoms and sought help? The more quickly you can get that pressure off the spinal cord, whether through surgery or anti-inflammatory drugs, the less likely any damage will be permanent. If you waited too long, investing in surgery may not be practical.

Location of the Disc

It may surprise you to learn that dogs with neck disc problems are, all things being equal, *more* likely to recover full function. Those cervical vertebrae are larger, so they allow a little more room for spinal cord swelling without permanent damage.

Walking or Not Walking?

Whether or not your dog can walk is an important element of your decision about whether to pursue surgery or crate rest. One of our favorite surgeons, who has a special interest in canine spinal biomechanics, says, "I don't like to cut a walking IVDD dog." If your dog is able to walk, many vets recommend that you start out with the conservative treatment and consider surgery only if the dog loses that ability or otherwise worsens.

Still Got Deep Pain Sensation?

Many vets believe that a dog who still has deep pain sensation has a greater chance of recovering the ability to walk after surgery. Some vets say that once a dog has lost deep pain sensation in the rear legs, surgery is more likely to be successful if performed within 24 hours. Others say that 24 hours is not a hard deadline.

Type/Severity of Disc Issue

Is the disc material swollen, or has it actually ruptured? Is the disc material pressing on the spinal cord (sometimes called a compression), or did it actually smack into the spinal cord with some speed (sometimes called a percussion)? If it was a percussion, did a plug actually penetrate the spinal cord like a bullet? All these questions affect the likelihood that your dachshund will walk again, whether you choose surgery or crate rest.

(It is not possible to know the type of disc issue without doing the pre-surgical imaging.)

Cost

Cost, of course, is a major consideration for many people. The cost of surgery can be a deal breaker, but don't assume you can't afford it. Surgery costs can range hugely from surgeon to surgeon and in different areas of the country.[1] Your dog's surgery may not be as expensive as you've heard from others. The cost of medications needed for eight weeks of crate rest will vary, of course, depending on the specific medications prescribed and the weight of your dog. A very rough estimate range is $100 to $250 for the eight-week period of crate rest.

How to Ask for an IVDD Surgery Cost Estimate

Ask your veterinarian for 2-3 referral surgeon options.

When you call, say this: "Hello, I'm trying to figure out whether surgery for my dog's IVDD is even a possibility for me. I know these things are really hard to estimate, and that there are a lot of factors, but can you tell me the standard cost at your facility for imaging (myelogram, CT scan, or MRI), a single-disc hemilaminectomy, and a week of hospitalization, assuming no complications?"

Some hospitals will not be comfortable giving an estimate this way. That's okay. It's worth a try.

[1] The Dodgerslist website maintains a list of surgery costs as reported by their members, generally ranging from $2,500 to $5,000. Some areas of the country range higher; others range lower.

what to expect with surgery

If you decide that surgery is your first choice for treating your dachshund's IVDD, your regular vet will give you a referral for a specialist surgeon. Here's what will happen next.

The surgeon needs to confirm the likely diagnosis of IVDD and locate as precisely as possible which disc is causing problems. To do this, they need to repeat some of the neurological exams (the pushing and pulling and pinching) that your regular vet did, and maybe do some new ones, looking for pain responses and reflexes.

After the exam, the surgeon will tell you whether IVDD is still the likely culprit, and whether imaging (myelogram, CT scan, or MRI) in preparation for surgery is recommended. The imaging tool gives the doctor an accurate picture of the discs and the spinal cord before doing any cutting. Any of these tools requires putting your dachshund under anesthesia.

Making the Imaging Decision

If you say *yes* to imaging, you are also giving a tentative *yes* to surgery. The surgeon will give you an estimate of the total cost, including hospitalization, and probably ask for a deposit. You will then go home and wait for the results.

If you no longer think surgery is the right way to go, for whatever reason, there is no point in getting the imaging. Just pay the consultation fee and be on your way. You're back to square one. You can still do conservative treatment with crate rest. Ask either vet to support you with the medications you need, starting now.

After Imaging: Making the Final Surgery Decision

When the imaging has given your surgeon a better picture of what is going on in your dachshund's spinal cord, they will step away from your unconscious dachshund to call you for a go/no-go decision about the surgery itself. You need to be ready to make this choice, because you have to make it right then and there, with the surgeon trying not to breathe impatiently in your ear through the phone and the surgical mask.

The surgeon will tell you which discs are affected and the type of disc problem, and probably a percentage likelihood of recovering the ability to walk. This is the last piece of information you will receive to decide whether or not surgery is indeed your best choice. If the answer is *yes*, give the surgeon the go-ahead and prepare for a few hours of worry.

what to expect with crate rest

If you believe that crate rest may be the best option for your dog and family, you need to understand how to do it right so you can make this decision with confidence.

> Whether your dog is paralyzed from IVDD, experiencing its excruciating pain, or having a less severe flare-up, the process for crate rest is the same.

During crate rest, you have only two jobs:

1. Provide a safe space and enough time for your dog to heal.
2. Control pain.

Crate Rest Job One: Provide a Safe Space and Enough Time to Heal.

Space is a crate. Time is eight weeks. The experience of many, many people has shown that the more you vary from those two simple understandings of those two simple terms, the less you will actually be doing your job: providing space and time to heal.

The Space: A Crate

A crate is a small cage, available at any pet supply store. The purpose of the crate is to keep your dog still enough that her spinal cord can heal, the pain can stop, and the signals from her brain can get through to her body again. Any time she moves around, healing can be slowed or reversed. Choose a crate that is just big enough for her to turn around in, but not so small that she is cramped up. She should be able to lie down on her side and stretch out with her legs out in front of her. Look for a crate with the wider side door or a top door—it will be easier to lift your dog in and out of that type. If your dog is a burrower, provide plenty of blankets to snuggle under for good rest.

The Time: Eight Weeks

You will read and hear differing opinions on the need for eight full weeks. People hold a lot of different views about the necessity of the eight full weeks.

We believe in the eight-week timeframe because IVDD is sneaky, and your dachshund is a Machiavellian genius. Together, they make a powerful, manipulative team. At some point during crate rest, your dachshund will start to feel better. As the swelling in her spinal cord goes down, her neurological signals will start to flow again. If she was paralyzed, she may start to stand up on her own. She will want out of the crate, and she will pull all her little tricks out of her little dachshund bag to get what she wants.

But even though her symptoms may have improved, that disc, with its weak spot, will still be in the process of healing. The weak spot is still weak. The IVDD is laying low like a serpent, egging her on, taking its diabolical time, looking for its opportunity to strike.

That's when IVDD is at its most cruel. Just as you think it might be safe to let her out of the crate, IVDD will rear up and gotcha! You'll have to start all over. The healing wasn't complete, so IVDD will seize its chance and come screaming back with a vengeance, like one of those ambushing Orcs from *Lord of the Rings*.

That's why we believe the full eight weeks is important.

If at any time during crate rest your dog's condition worsens, you will need to go back to the vet immediately to reassess what to do.

Crate Rest Job Two: Control Pain.

This job is about drugs. You *must* have drugs. You need at least two drugs, probably three, maybe four, and possibly five.

1. An anti-inflammatory to reduce the swelling and pressure on the spinal cord. It also contributes to relieving some pain.
2. A second pain medication, and maybe two, for breakthrough pain.
3. A tummy soother, especially if your anti-inflammatory drug is a steroid.
4. A muscle relaxant.
5. A sedative (for the dog, not you—ask your own doctor for one for yourself).

Don't worry. Specifics are on page 46. These drugs are widely available and should not be expensive.

Backup Plan. You also want to talk to your vet about what to do if your dog's pain is not controlled at a time when the vet office is closed (after hours or on a weekend). Be sure to find an emergency veterinary hospital you can access if needed.

some final thoughts on choosing a treatment

What works for one dog may not work at all for another dog. What worked for one dog this time may not work for the same dog the next time. There are too many variables to definitively predict an outcome of either treatment, especially without imaging or actually cutting the dog open and seeing what there is to see.

Only surgery actually removes the ruptured disc material that is pressing on the cord (if, in fact, the disc has actually ruptured). If you choose crate rest, you are banking on the body's ability to reabsorb or redistribute that disc material before permanent damage has been done. Soft disc material may reabsorb, but hard pieces (like the disc coating) may not.

Before assuming that you cannot pay for surgery, make sure you know what the surgery is likely to cost in your area, and exhaust all your options for getting help with the costs (family, friends, fundraising).

If you cannot provide surgery, crate rest is a viable option. It is at least a chance.

And remember, even if neither treatment path works, your dog can still have a happy life. It will be a different life, but it can still be a happy one for both of you.

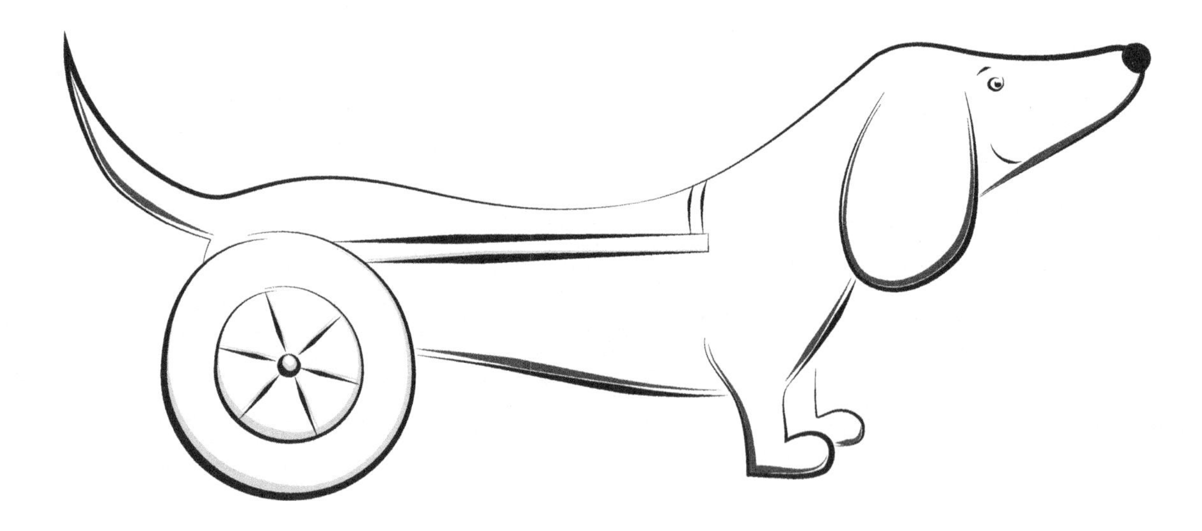

honey, have you squeezed the dachshund?

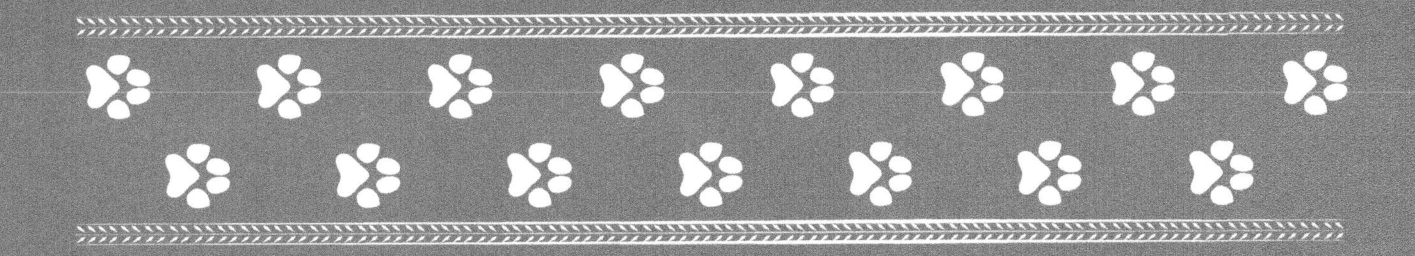

In the following sections, you will find a great deal more detail on all of the topics we have gone over, as well as preventing an IVDD injury, living with the condition, and (should your treatment not restore function), caring for a down dog.

decision 1:

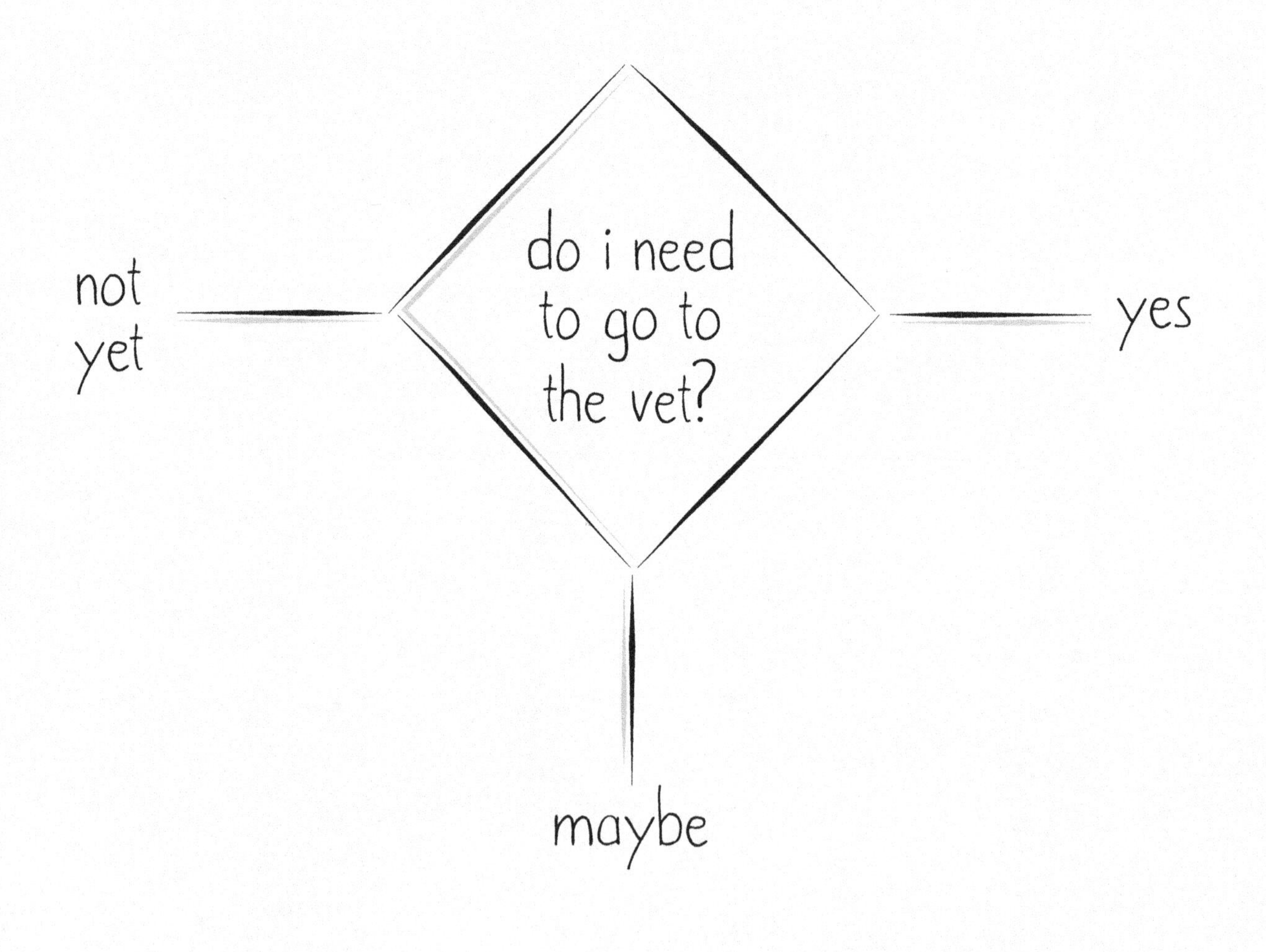

part one: i think my dog has had an IVDD injury. what should i do?

There is something you need to hear: you have a lot of options available to you, more than you think. But one thing is not an option: doing nothing. An IVDD flare-up is agonizing. It is painful and terrifying for your dachshund. You must take some kind of action to help, and you must do that action right away. To ignore what is happening, or to withhold treatment, is cruel. Your dog is suffering, and you are the one—the only one—who has control over the situation.

You're going to have to pull up those big girl (or big boy) panties. You're going to have to deal.

As soon as you suspect IVDD, you need to make two main decisions fairly quickly. The first decision is *Do I need to go to the veterinarian?* The second decision is one of two questions: *If it is IVDD, what kind of treatment am I going to use?* Or maybe, *if it is IVDD and I decide not to treat it, what will I do instead?*

Let's look at each decision and what you need to think about as you make it.

Decision 1: Do I Need to Go to the Veterinarian?

The short answer: yes. You need veterinary help, especially if this is your first time dealing with suspected IVDD in this dog. Your dachshund needs pain relief and prescription medication, and you need a definitive diagnosis. You can't get these without a medical professional's support.

The longer answer: maybe. After you and this dog have dealt with IVDD once, you may not need to go to the vet every single time your dog has an issue.

If you decide not to go to the vet, be ready to flex your decision as things go along. If your dog starts out in pain but is not paralyzed and you have the medications, going straight to crate rest is a reasonable choice. But if you cannot manage pain or you see loss of function, reconsider going to the veterinarian. In fact, be ready to reconsider at any time, depending on what happens.

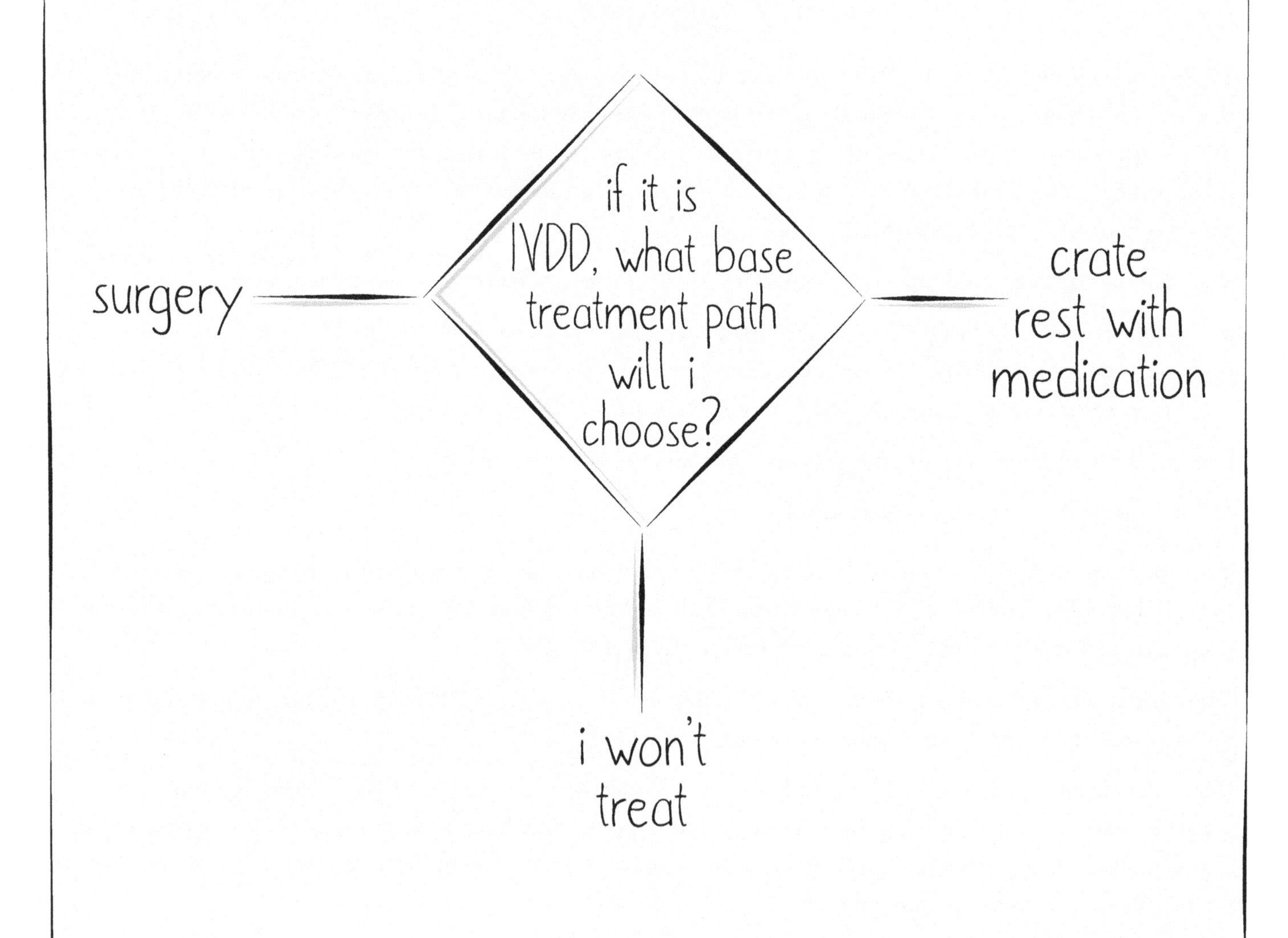
decision 2:
if it is IVDD, what base treatment path will i choose?
surgery
crate rest with medication
i won't treat

But really, the answer is yes. Go to the vet. Especially if your dog cannot walk or is exhibiting signs of constant and terrible pain, in which case, please go to the vet. Emergency vet, if necessary.

> If you have all of these...
>
> - Experience with IVDD with this dog
> - Medications on hand that will reduce swelling and manage pain
> - A reasonable level of confidence that you really are dealing with a disc flare-up
>
> ...then you don't need to rush to the vet. At least, not at first.

Decision 2: If It Is IVDD, What Kind of Treatment Am I Going to Use?

Your treatment choice must solve two problems for your dog:

1. Relieve the pain.
2. Relieve the pressure on the spinal cord.

To solve these two problems, you have two basic approaches available:[2] surgery, or crate rest with meds (conservative treatment).

Other therapies exist, of course. Some common ones are laser therapy, acupuncture, chiropractic treatment, holistic therapies, physical therapy, swim therapy, and various supplements and injections. Our experience has been that these therapies are not useful unless you also do either surgery or crate rest. Some could even be harmful at this stage.

If you decide not to treat the IVDD flare-up, you can read about your choices under "The Four Non-Treatment Options" on page 58.

[2] Veterinary researchers all over the world are working on other treatment options, but these are the two main options we have available now.

the vet exam

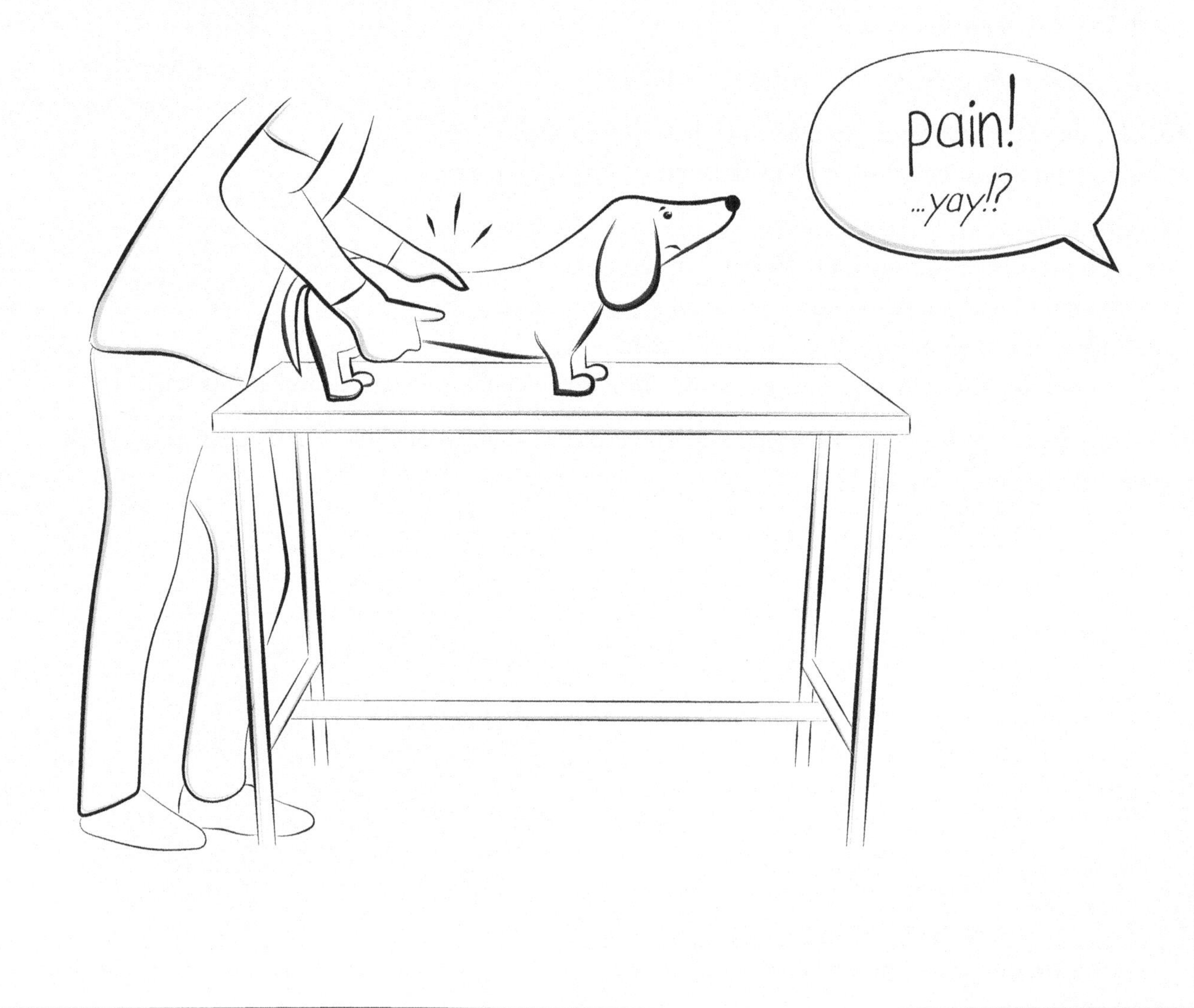

the vet exam: what can i expect?

Your veterinarian will start by performing a basic examination. They will be looking for signs and symptoms of other conditions or injuries, just in case IVDD is not your culprit.

> **I Hear Hoofbeats...**
>
> If you are bringing in a dachshund with a painful back, one of your vet's top suspicions should immediately be IVDD because of the frequency with which it occurs in dachshunds.[3] As they say, "when you hear hoofbeats, think horses, not zebras."
>
> Of course, your dog could have something besides IVDD, but IVDD should always be top of mind with a dachshund.

After the basic exam, your vet's likely next step will be some hands-on neurological tests. These tests involve a lot of pushing, pulling, prodding, and pinching. Parts of the exam can be painful, but you *want* to see evidence of pain. Pain means that at least some neurological signals are getting through. It will feel very odd to rejoice when things cause your dachshund to hurt, but if you see a response to painful stimuli, give a quiet little celebratory holler and praise your dog. *Try to keep a positive attitude for your dachshund, who will be frightened and looking to you for cues on how to react.*

All this pinching and pulling gives the veterinarian information about whether and how to diagnose IVDD. When a dog loses motor function, that loss happens in a specific order: proprioception (your dog's ability to correct her footing), shallow pain sensation (think skin pinch or bug bite), and then deep pain sensation (nerves deep in the tissue). The exam will tell your veterinarian where on this continuum your dog falls. It also provides a pretty good idea of where on the spine the problem sits.

[3] IVDD occurs in only 2% of the general dog population, but about 25% of dachshunds.

You will probably see your veterinarian figuring out the answers to these questions:

- How does your dog stand, balance, and move?
- Does she correct her footing if I curl her toes under, or do her feet stay knuckled under?
- Does the skin on her back twitch if I pinch the top layer of skin all along the backbone?
- If I use the little mallet (like the school nurse used to do), will her reflexes contract the right muscles or tendons?
- Does she pull her tail back down when I lift it?
- Is her anus puckered or loose? Does it react to being touched?
- If I pinch (hard! with a clamp!) between the toes, does she pull her foot back?
- Does she react to any of this by looking surprised, turning her head, or crying out?

After all of that, the veterinarian may want to do an x-ray. X-rays cannot definitively diagnose IVDD, but they are still useful—they can rule out other things (like a fracture or a vertebral tumor). In some cases, a veterinarian will see abnormal-looking narrow spaces between vertebrae, a strong indication of IVDD. Sometimes a vet will see calcifications of the discs, but these are not proof of IVDD and may not be the actual cause of, or even the location for, your dog's immediate pain and symptoms.[4]

If the vet wants to do bloodwork, find out why. Bloodwork is a treasure chest of information, but it does not tell us much about diagnosing IVDD. If your veterinarian wants bloodwork, they probably suspect something besides IVDD or have concerns about your dog's ability to tolerate surgery or the medications needed for conservative treatment.[5]

With all of this information, your veterinarian should now be able to tell you whether IVDD has joined your family as the most unwanted houseguest ever.

---

[4] Calcifications are one of the great IVDD mysteries.

[5] Bloodwork is generally recommended before surgery to gauge a dog's likely ability to handle anesthesia. Your vet might also want the bloodwork to make sure that the liver and kidneys are able to handle some of the medications often used for crate rest.

the neurological exam

From the Desk of Dr. Christman

When I perform a neurological exam, I get a significant amount of information about whether to diagnose IVDD and how to recommend treatment. The neurological tests most related to IVDD are posture and gait, proprioceptive placing, panniculus reflex, patellar reflex, gastrocnemius reflex, withdrawal reflex, perineal reflex, and deep pain response.

Some patients have too much pain to tolerate the tests. In these cases, I may administer a light narcotic (like buprenorphine) to make them comfortable enough for the exam while still allowing me to observe pain responses. Testing these reflexes and responses helps me understand how severe the problem is and what course of action to recommend. For example, if your dog's back feet do not knuckle over on themselves, and she withdraws her legs when I squeeze on her toes, that tells me that there is likely an inflammation at the disc versus a complete IVDD rupture. She may be able to recover with strict rest, medications, and frequent re-checks.

The exam also helps me to neurolocalize, or identify where on the spine the problem originates. Could it be between C1-C5? Maybe C6-T2? T3-L3? L4-S4? For example, a dog who can walk, but who acts "drunk" in the back legs with exaggerated patellar and femoral reflexes, probably has an issue in the mid-thoracic (T) to lumbar (L) region.

Many general practitioners use x-rays when they suspect IVDD. An x-ray can eliminate other possibilities like spinal tumors, but it will not show the spinal cord or discs themselves. An x-ray can show indirect evidence of disc lesions. Sometimes we can see a divot, or narrowing of the spaces between the vertebrae, as the disc material crowds them. Vets call this the loss of "horsehead appearance," since the normal vertebrae look like the heads of horses on radiographs.

If I suspect a paralyzed dog has IVDD, I generally do not perform spinal x-rays, especially if my client is expense-conscious. That's where additional diagnostics come in to play. I would rather have my pet owners invest their finances in more sensitive diagnostic imaging tools, such as an MRI or CT scan, that can actually show us what is happening with the spinal cord and discs.

—Adam Christman, DVM, MBA

Cs, Ts, and Ls

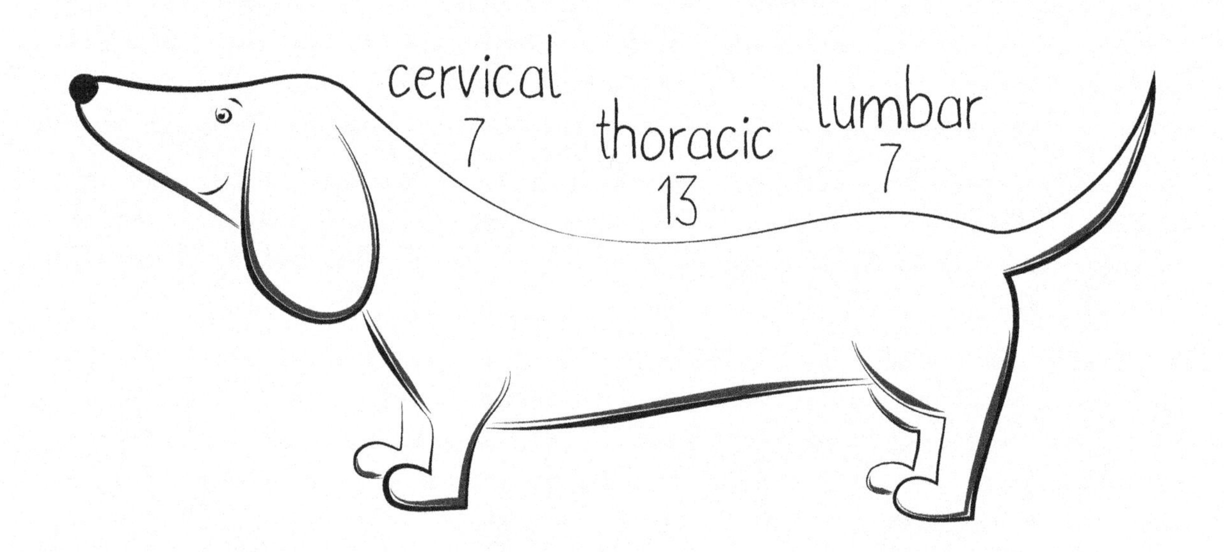

know your Cs, Ts, and Ls

When you talk to people whose dogs have IVDD, it won't be long until you hear them tossing around the letters C, T, and L as if they were veterinarians themselves. Don't be intimidated; you will soon be speaking this language too. C, T, and L are just the codes vets use to describe where a disc problem is:

- C stands for cervical—the discs in the neck.
- T refers to the discs in the middle of the back—the thoracic discs.
- L is for lumbar, the lowest discs down by the tail.

Each disc is identified with the letter that describes its region and the numbers of the vertebrae that it sits between. So if your veterinarian says that your dog's disc problem is at C3-C4, they're talking about the disc between the third and fourth vertebrae in the neck; if they say T6-T7, the problem is about halfway down the back in the thoracic region; and so on.

Disc Stats

About 65 percent of all disc ruptures are in the T region (middle of the back), while cervical (neck) discs account for about 18 percent of disc ruptures. I'll let you do the math on what that means for the L discs.

how do you decide?

From the Desk of Dr. Christman

After I diagnose a dog with IVDD, I generally recommend one of two courses of action.

For a dog who is not paralyzed and can urinate on her own, I prescribe steroids, muscle relaxants, and other pain medications as needed. I instruct the family to closely confine the dog for several weeks, and we schedule several check-ins so that we can make sure recovery is progressing as it should.

Obviously, I take a dog who is paralyzed very seriously, and I recommend quick action if my diagnosis is IVDD. I am a general practitioner, so I refer these patients to a specialist for possible surgery: the nearest specialist or the teaching hospital at a veterinary school.

Time is not on your side. With a disc rupture, the quicker we act, the more likely we are to avoid permanent damage. In a matter of hours, a dog with IVDD can lose conscious proprioception, superficial pain sensation, and deep pain sensation, in that order. After deep pain sensation is lost, surgery is less likely to work. A patient who is able to have surgery should do so as soon as possible to give her the best possible chance of walking again.

If I believe that surgery gives a dog the highest likelihood of recovering the ability to walk, it can be difficult for me to advise another course of action. Surgery is not cheap, but it is the quickest way to take that pressure off the spinal cord.

If surgery is just not in the cards, we talk about medical management: strict crate rest with medications. I believe that a veterinarian must be brutally honest about prognosis, so I make sure that my owners know there is a good chance that their dog may be permanently paralyzed. On the other hand, I also inform people about the high quality of life a dog can have even if permanently disabled. My Cosmo is certainly a happy guy!

—Adam Christman, DVM, MBA

part two: base treatment details

what to expect with IVDD surgery

You've decided that surgery is your first choice for treating your dachshund's IVDD. Your regular veterinarian gave you a referral to a specialty hospital that houses either a surgeon or neurologist. You're taking all your deepest breaths. You're checking your account balances online, and you think that if you cancel cable for a few months and pack peanut butter sandwiches for lunch, you can pull it off. And there's always your birthday money from Great Aunt Mildred. With some stretching and some begging and some creative fundraising, you can make this work. Somehow.

Here's what will happen next.

The exam—*again.*

The surgeon needs to confirm the likely diagnosis of IVDD and locate as closely as possible which disc is causing problems. To do this, they will repeat some of the neurological tests your regular veterinarian did, and maybe do some new ones. They will be looking for pain responses and reflexes.

That's right: the pulling and pinching all over again. You've seen this routine once, and it wasn't pleasant the first time, so this may be frustrating and difficult to watch. There will be times that you will want to shriek, "Get on with it!" *Remember that your dachshund will be frightened, in pain, and looking to you for cues. Keep your voice and your body language positive. No screaming or curling up in the fetal position until you're in the parking lot where your dog cannot see and hear you.*

After the exam, the surgeon will tell you whether they still think IVDD is the likely culprit and whether an imaging tool is recommended to get a more accurate picture of what is happening with the discs and spinal cord. This is your next decision point.

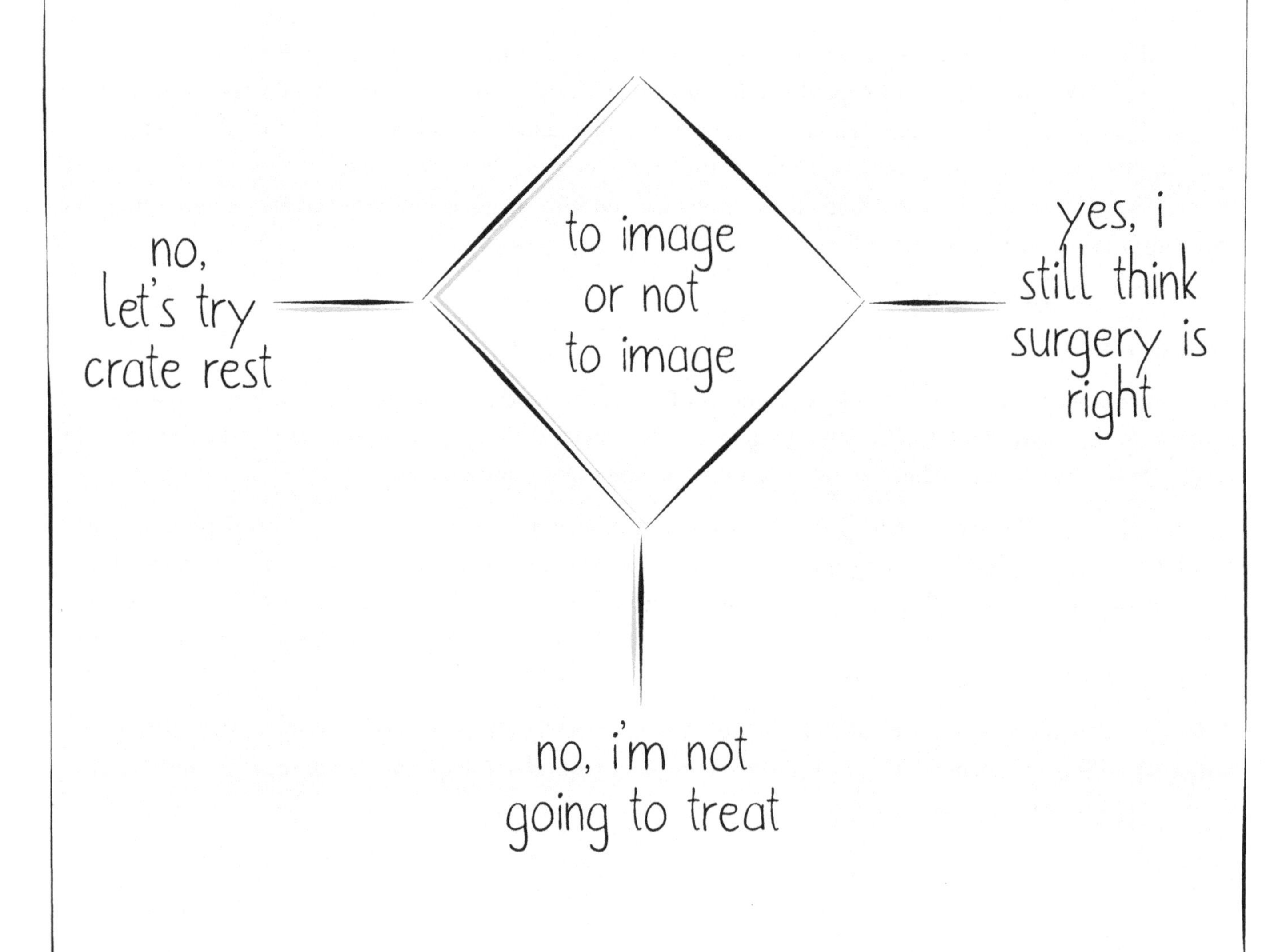
decision 3:
to image
or not
to image
no,
let's try
crate rest
yes, i
still think
surgery is
right
no, i'm not
going to treat

Decision 3: To Image, or Not to Image?

The surgeon needs to use an imaging tool (myelogram, CT scan, or MRI[6]) to get an accurate picture of the discs and spinal cord before doing any cutting. Any of these tools requires putting your dachshund under anesthesia. At some facilities, it also requires scheduling the equipment. Imaging is not a willy-nilly thing that vets can do on a whim, like an x-ray. This equipment is not something the techs fool around with at the holiday party.

If you say *yes* to imaging, you are also giving a tentative *yes* to surgery.[7] Your surgeon will give you an estimate of the total cost (including imaging and hospitalization), and they may ask for a deposit. They will probably tell you to go home and wait for The Phone Call. Slap down the plastic, whisper to your little one that you'll see her tomorrow, and head back to the house.

You'll feel profoundly unresolved.

the phone call

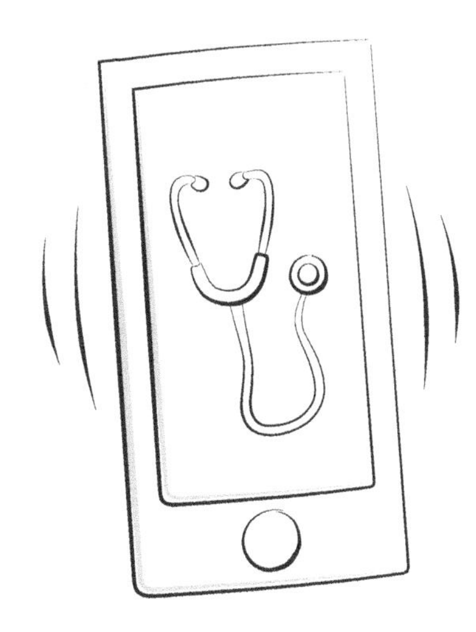

When the imaging has given your surgeon a better picture of what is going on in your dachshund's spinal cord, they will step away from your unconscious dachshund to call you for a go/no go decision about the surgery itself. You need to be ready to make this choice, because you have to make it right then and there, with the surgeon trying not to breathe impatiently in your ear through the phone and surgical mask.

Why do you have to decide so fast? For one, your dachshund is under anesthesia. If you want your dachshund to have surgery, you want to put her under only once. And you want to minimize the time the disc presses on the spinal cord (and potentially damages it). In other words, it's *showtime.*

[6] See the Glossary on page 128 for a description of each of these tests.

[7] If you no longer think surgery is the right way to go (for whatever reason), there is no point in getting the imaging. Just pay the consultation fee and be on your way. You're back to square one. You can still do conservative treatment with crate rest. Ask either vet to support you with the medications you need, starting right away. Use the checklist in the Crate Rest section on page 48 to make sure you are ready.

> **Be Ready**
>
> You need to be ready to process the information that the surgeon gives you very quickly. So it's best, as much as possible, to work your way through all the emotional and financial parts of deciding which way to go before the surgeon calls.
>
> See the worksheet on the next page.

During The Phone Call, the surgeon will tell you which discs are affected and the type of disc problem. They will also give you The Percentage—a likelihood of recovering the ability to walk.[8]

The Percentage will loom large in your mind, but remember two things about it:

1. The Percentage is difficult to estimate. Many variables are involved.
2. The Percentage is even more difficult to estimate when you consider that some dachshunds do not start to walk until weeks or months after surgery.

While The Percentage is a big component of your choice, it is not the only one. As you wait for The Phone Call, reflect on your emotions and the different elements of your decision, using the worksheet questions on the following page as guidance. This is a lot to process, and unfortunately, there is no formula to calculate the right answer. Much depends on your situation and your values. But with the answers to these questions and some careful thought, you can make a compassionate, well-informed decision.

The worksheet can be downloaded from our website or Facebook pages.

[8] If the imaging showed something other than IVDD, the vet will tell you that. Then you need a different book.

YOUR THOUGHTS ABOUT SURGERY

What chance of regaining function (The Percentage) do I need to hear to go forward with surgery? (Be realistic, but honest.)	
How important is The Percentage in my decision?	
If I don't get at least The Percentage that I want, do I want to try crate rest with meds?	
With what I know now about disabled dachshunds and their quality of life, am I willing to get on with a new life with a disabled dog if that is the outcome of all of this?	

SUGGESTED QUESTIONS TO ASK THE SURGEON DURING THE PHONE CALL

Question	Surgeon's Answer
What did you see? Was it IVDD?	
Which discs were affected?	
Did you see a rupture?	
Did the rupture look like it was penetrating like a plug or bullet?	
Did you see any evidence of damage to the spinal cord?	
Will the surgery relieve her pain, even if she doesn't regain the ability to walk?	
What is your estimated likelihood of recovering full ability to walk and control the bladder? (This is The Percentage. Don't ask for 100%. You're not going to get it.)	
Do you expect recovery to happen right after surgery or with some time?	
What is the surgical procedure that you will use called?	
Will there be fenestration (will you cut a window in the spine)?	
Has the estimated cost changed?	
How long do you expect post-surgical care to last? What will that be like?	

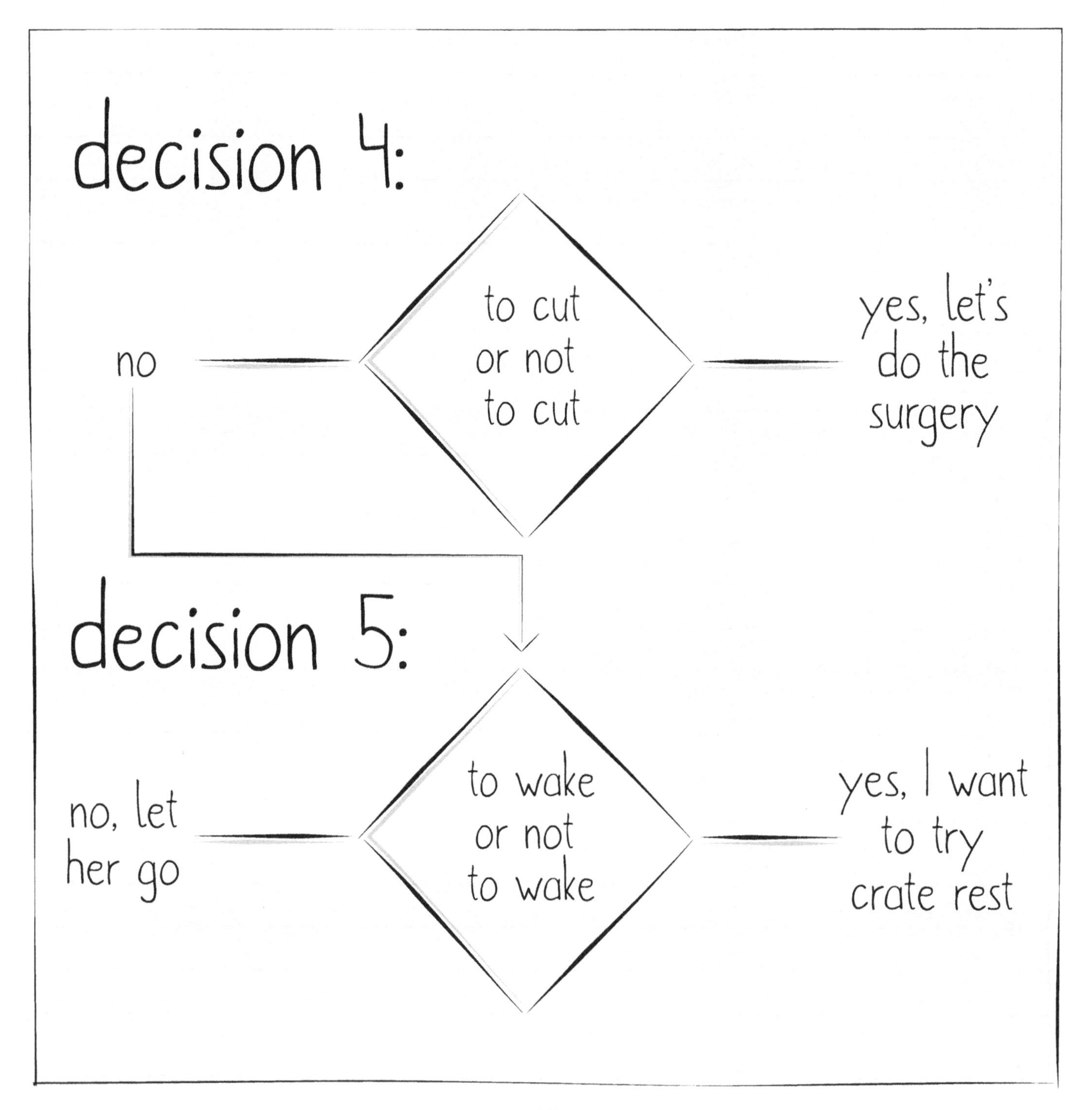
decision 4:
no
to cut
or not
to cut
yes, let's
do the
surgery
decision 5:
no, let
her go
to wake
or not
to wake
yes, I want
to try
crate rest

Decision 4: To Cut, or Not To Cut?

With the imaging, you have the last piece of information you need in order to decide whether or not surgery is indeed your best choice.

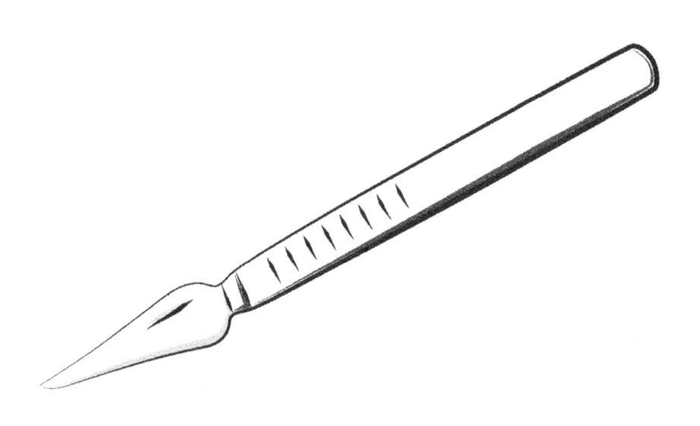

- If the answer is *yes*, give the surgeon the go-ahead and prepare for a few hours of worry.
- If the imaging results changed your mind about surgery, you have yet another difficult choice to make. (This is the last one for a little while, I promise.)

Decision 5: To Wake, or Not To Wake?

If you decide against surgery, you must choose between waking your dachshund up and trying crate rest with meds, or letting her go while she is still under anesthesia.

If you decide to try crate rest, you may need to emphasize to the surgeon (and to your regular veterinarian) that you have accepted that your dachshund may be permanently disabled. You understand what disability involves, and you are willing to live with that choice. You want to try the conservative treatment, and you need their support with the medications needed to manage pain and reduce inflammation.

If you decide to let her go, you can do so knowing that you did everything possible to give her a strong chance. You educated yourself. You thought about all your options, and you considered all the different facets of each option. You thought about a dog's life with less than full abilities. IVDD is cruel, and sometimes it refuses to be denied. Many, many people have walked this painful road before you, and many will walk it after. You did all of this with love and compassion, and you decided to spare her additional pain and confusion with little chance of reaching a pain-free state.

Please reach out to one or more of the Supportive Communities listed in the Resources to connect with people who will understand what you've been through.

After Surgery

More than likely, your little one's surgery stay will last for a few days (most dogs stay at the hospital for about a week). Hospitals encourage you to visit during that time. Visit as often as you can, and keep up that positive attitude for your dog. The swelling from the surgery itself (separate from the swelling due to the disc rupture) can take two full weeks to go down. This can be extremely frustrating (not to mention frightening and heartbreaking). You may not see any progress until then.

The first time you visit, things may not look very good. She will probably be wrapped in a pee pad and have gauze taped over her back. She may be propped up in her cage with rolled towels to stabilize the spine. She probably will not look happy. She may look the opposite of happy: very, very pitiful. You may doubt the whole decision—including your ability to be objective, your thought process, whether you were being selfish, all of it.

But, stop for a moment and consider what that surgery involved! Your dog's back was cut open, bone cut away, her spinal cord exposed, and disc gunk cleaned out. Of course she's not going to spring back immediately. A lot of stuff went down in that operating room, with some very sensitive body parts. It's completely understandable that she would look awful at this point. Don't be discouraged.

Pain management immediate post-surgery can be a struggle. Some dogs will need a pain patch, which gradually releases a powerful pain medication. These drugs often make dogs woozy or confused.

The day will come when the surgeon says, "Tomorrow, she can go home." And you might be a little afraid, because then, you realize, it's going to be up to you. That can be daunting. Preparing for your dachshund's convalescence after surgery is a lot like preparing for crate rest; please look at the table to the right for tips.

When You Go to Pick Her Up

Bring your crate into the surgeon's office so you can put your dog right into it and carry her in the crate to the car. When you arrive at the surgeon for Go Home Day, your dog will either be able to walk, or she won't. She will either be able to pee without help, or she won't. If she can walk and pee independently, that's terrific. But lack of function after a week isn't necessarily a reason to give up hope that your dog will regain those abilities. Give these things some time. Give them some effort. Try very hard—very, very hard—to keep up hope. It can take days, or even weeks, for function to come back. Sadly, a very common time that people euthanize a dog is when the surgery didn't work right away.

Every surgeon has a post-surgery protocol for resting, controlling pain, troubleshooting, and starting rehab. Expect to keep your dog confined for a while, especially when you aren't at home. You want to prevent any movements that have an impact on the back. The disc itself takes time to heal, and you don't want another rupture out of that weak spot. You also need to make sure that your dachshund doesn't gnaw at any stitches or staples. As the incision heals, it will itch.

Don't be reluctant to ask your veterinarian for leeway in managing pain—your dachshund shouldn't have to endure pain during this period. Ask what drugs you can give, and ask how much more often you can give them, if your dog seems upset or in pain. Ask what you should do if it gets bad in the middle of the night.

Before you head home, ask the surgeon how long you should restrict her activity and when you can begin physical rehabilitation, such as passive range of motion exercises, stretching, brushing, balancing, towel or sling walking, and swimming, if needed.

We Did the Surgery, Now What?

Some dogs come out of surgery ready to rock and roll, and they never look back. Other dogs' surgeries do not completely restore the ability to walk, or at least not right away. And many dogs come out of surgery with swelling that can take up to two weeks to subside. Ask your surgeon when your dog can resume activity and start serious rehabilitation, whether at-home, DIY rehab or at a veterinary rehab center. Be clear about the therapies you are considering (especially weight-bearing techniques or anything that manipulates the spine itself). See "Do We Need More Rehab?" on page 68 for some possibilities.

If you went to the expense and effort to get surgery for your dog, your hopes were probably high, regardless of the odds your surgeon gave you. Then you went to pick up your dog. Maybe she wasn't walking. In fact, she looked pretty terrible. There was a Frankenstein scar with staples (and it was much longer than you expected it to be). There may have been a pain patch. She probably looked miserable. And maybe your surgeon (who is a surgeon, after all, not a physical therapist) basically told you, "Best of luck, then!" and checked you out. And you left, carrying your little still-crippled dog in your arms, stunned and horrified and with no idea what to do (even though you might have been given a thick, slippery pile of papers, brochures, notes, educational sheets, and records about after-care to take home).

The surgeon's expertise is in removing the offending disc material and getting the spinal cord ready to heal. That's a surgeon's slice of the problem.

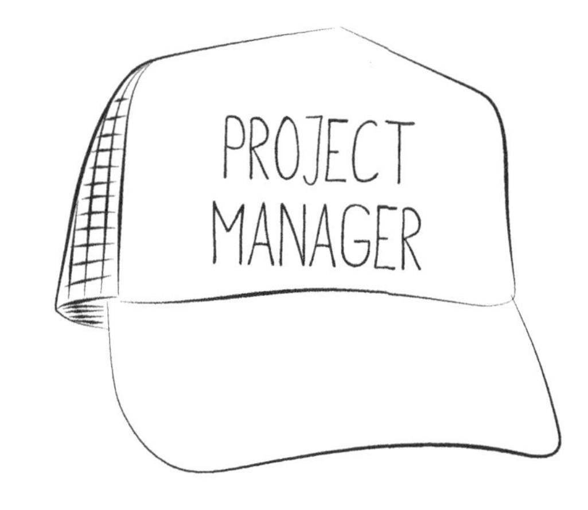

You are the project manager. Your slice of the problem is to be the general contractor. Once surgery is over, it's up to you to manage the process of your dog's recovery and all the people who might need to be involved. Many veterinarians and therapists believe that the more complementary therapies you do, the greater the chance that your dog will walk again. That's where the add-on therapies come in.

Typical Post-Surgery Convalescence

This protocol for taking care of your dog after surgery will give you an idea of what to expect (but be sure to follow your surgeon's instructions).

Week One	• You will need to protect the incision, but you probably will not need to do any actual wound care. • Week 1 will be taken up by making sure she stays comfortable, keeping up with the potty schedule, and watching out for reactions to the medications, like nausea or diarrhea. (See the Crate Rest Troubleshooting table on page 51 – post-surgery troubleshooting is very similar.) • You may need to squeeze the abdomen to encourage the bladder to urinate and stimulate under the tail to encourage the bowels to move. • Your surgeon may encourage you to start some gentle at-home exercises. • If you are interested in starting anti-inflammatory therapies, like laser or acupuncture, ask your surgeon if they have any concerns. • Most surgeons schedule a follow-up visit to check the wound and take out the stitches or staples in seven to ten days.
Weeks Two–Six	• Many surgeons advise limiting weight-bearing activity for six weeks to allow the disc coating to heal (and avoid another rupture), including walking, assisted or otherwise. • After the sutures come out, you may be able to start non-weight-bearing rehab, such as swim therapy. Ask your surgeon about this. • A resistance band under your dog's abdomen can help with walking to go outside to potty. The band also helps with learning to regain motor function. • Ask your surgeon about therapies like underwater treadmill, swimming, and acupuncture. • Gradually increase activity day by day. • Your surgeon will give you a schedule for doing different exercises at home about three or four times a day. See the next page for suggestions on building these into your routine.
After Week Six	• Surgery site and damaged discs should be strong enough for the Rehabilitation activities listed in "Do We Need More Rehab" on page 68, unless your surgeon or regular veterinarian advises otherwise.

Sample At-Home Exercises Schedule

When You...	You Can Also...
Take her outside to pee	• Do standing and balancing exercises • Do towel/sling walking (when balance improves and surgeon says weight-bearing is okay)
Watch TV in the mornings and evenings	• Squeeze and massage between her toes (for deep pain sensation) • Do passive range of motion on rear legs (to keep muscles toned and build strength) • Stretch rear legs (to keep muscles limber) • Have her stand on a pillow with both front and rear legs to help engage her core and regain balance • Massage the surgical site lightly to help break down scar tissue
Brush your teeth	• Do a quick brush of her legs (to stimulate nerve connections)

what to expect with crate rest

If you believe that crate rest (also known as conservative treatment or medical management) may be the best option for your dog and family, you need to understand how to do it correctly so that you can make this decision with confidence.

> The process for crate rest is the same, whether your dog is paralyzed from IVDD, experiencing its excruciating pain, or having a less severe flare-up.

During crate rest, you have only two jobs:

1. Provide a safe space and enough time for your dog to heal.
2. Control pain.

We will talk about each of these jobs and exactly what you need to do to give your dog the best chance of success with crate rest.

job 1: provide space and time to heal

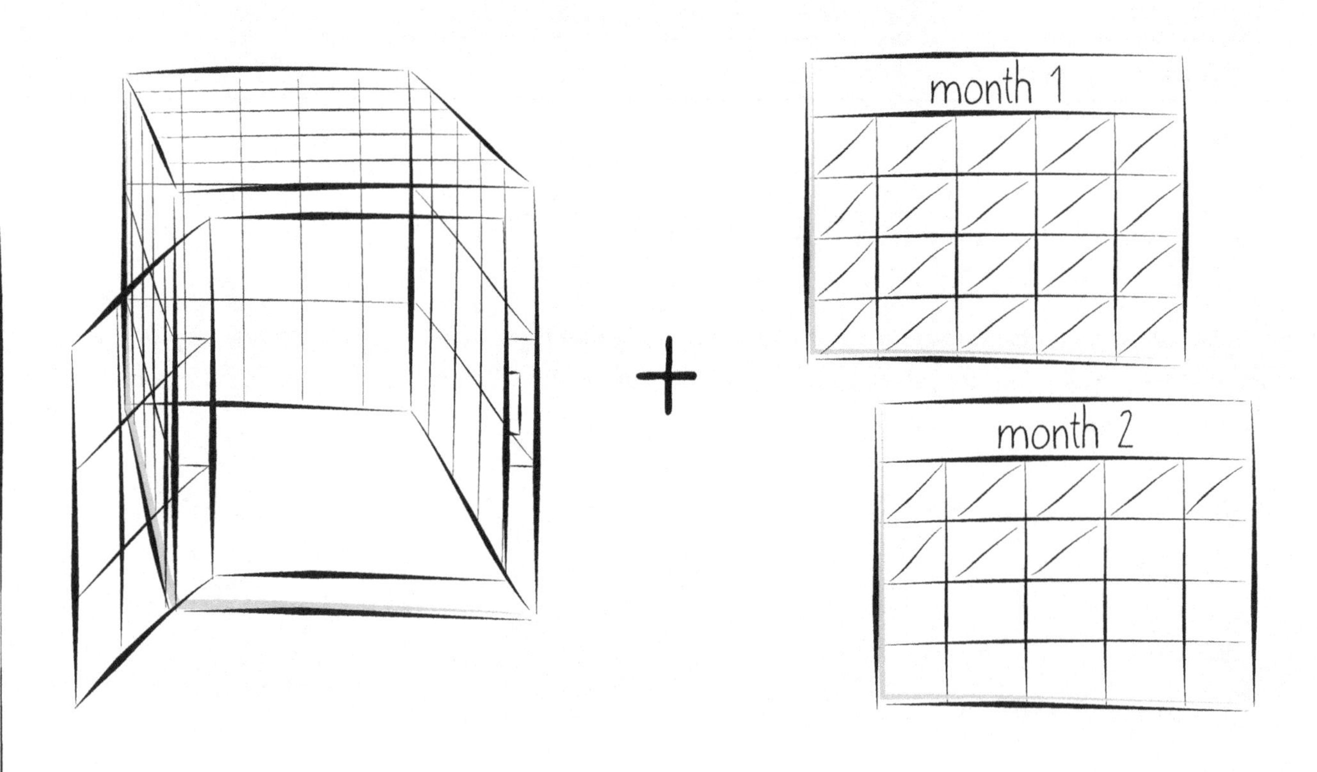

Job One: Provide a Safe Space and Enough Time to Heal

In the simplest, bluntest terms possible: Space is a crate. Time is eight weeks.

Before you start arguing about your special circumstances and why those terms should not apply to your dog, let's just agree up front that every dog is different, every home is different, and every family is different.

Yes, there are times when you will have to use your judgment on what safe space and enough time mean for you.

But the experience of many, many people has shown that the more you change those two simple understandings of those two simple terms, the less you will actually be doing your first job: providing space and time to heal.

I'm really sorry about this. I would change it if I could.

The Space: A Crate

A crate is a small cage, and it's available at any pet supply store. The purpose of the crate is to keep your dog still enough that her beautiful, fragile little spinal cord can heal, the pain can stop, and the signals from her brain can get through to her body again. Any time she moves around, jostling that disc in its earliest stages of healing, recovery can be slowed or reversed. The crate should be small: just big enough for her to turn around in, but not so small that she is cramped. She should be able to lie down on her side and stretch out with her legs in front of her. If possible, buy a crate with the wider side door—it will be easier to lift your dog in and out.

> Don't go buy a giant, bull mastiff-size crate and then tell yourself your dachshund is doing crate rest. That is following the letter of the law, not the spirit of it.
>
> That will not work.

The Time: Eight Weeks

Eight weeks. If you're in Spain, that's ocho semanas. France? Huit semaines. Germany? Acht weken. Japan? Hachi Shúkan. Get it? No matter where you are in the world, *eight weeks is eight weeks.*

You will read and hear differing opinions on the need for eight full weeks. Knowledgeable people, including veterinarians, hold a lot of different opinions about the necessity of the eight weeks.

I believe in the eight-week timeframe because IVDD is sneaky, and your dachshund is a Machiavellian genius. Together, they make a powerful, manipulative team. At some point during crate rest, if all goes well, your

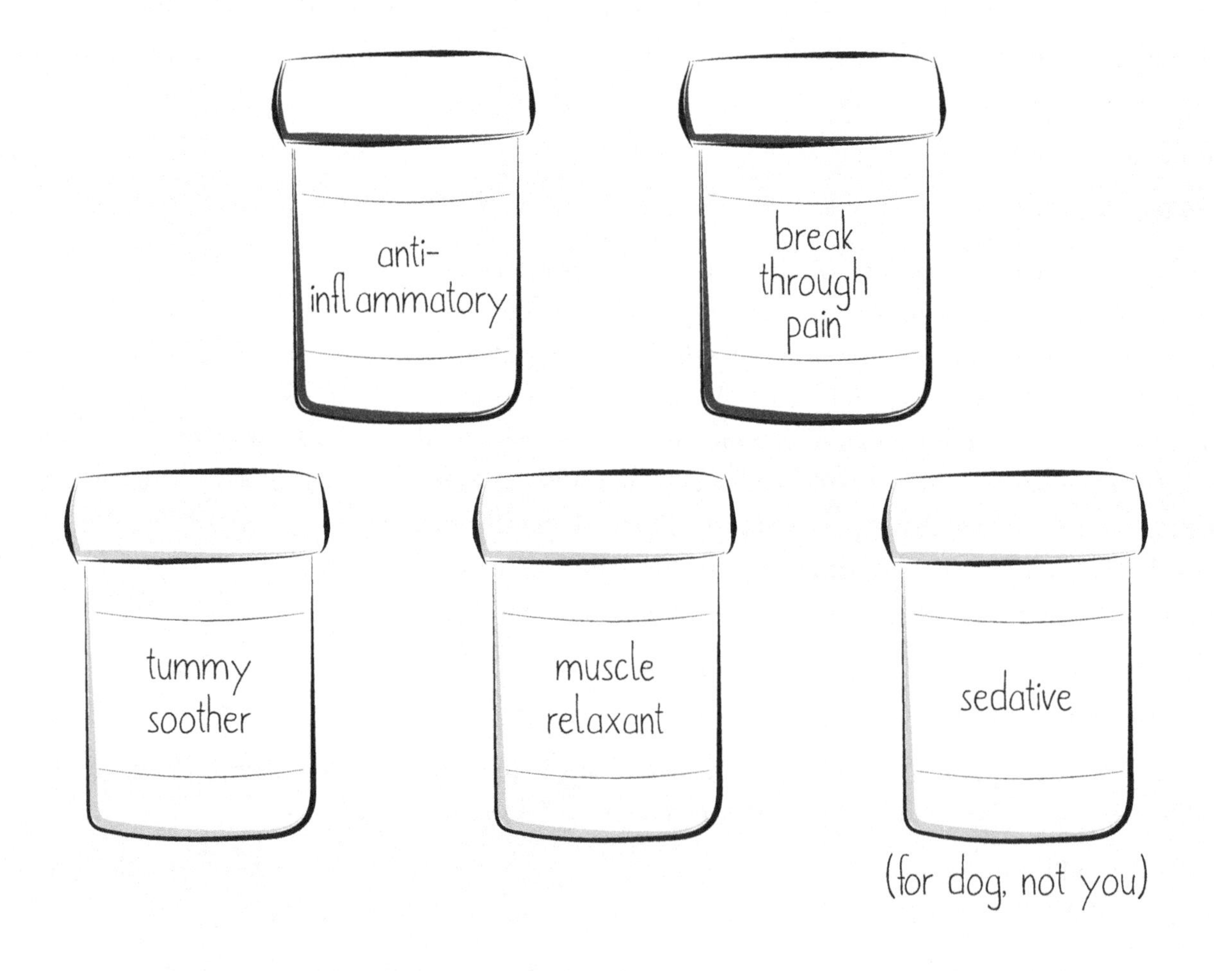
job 2: control pain
anti-
inflammatory
break
through
pain
tummy
soother
muscle
relaxant
sedative
(for dog, not you)

dachshund will start to feel better. As the swelling in her spinal cord goes down, her neurological signals will start to flow again. If she was paralyzed, she may start to stand up on her own. Thrillingly, her tail may wag! She will want out of the crate, and she will pull all her little tricks out of her little dachshund bag to get what she wants.

But even though her symptoms have improved, that disc, with its weak spot, is still in the process of healing. The weak spot is still weak. The IVDD is laying low like a serpent, egging her on, taking its diabolical time, looking for its opportunity to strike.

That's when IVDD is at its most cruel. Just when you think it might be safe to let her out of the crate, IVDD will rear up and gotcha! Up flares the pain again. Or down she goes again. You'll have to start all over. The healing wasn't complete, so IVDD will seize its chance to take advantage of that weak spot and come screaming back with a vengeance, like one of those ambushing Orcs from *Lord of the Rings*.

That's why I believe the eight weeks are important.

Job Two: Control Pain

After all that rigmarole about time and space and serpents and Orcs, you forgot you had another job, didn't you? But it's essential.

You must control pain.

This job is about drugs. You *must* have drugs, which means you must have a veterinarian. You need at least two drugs, probably three, maybe four, and possibly five. Maybe more! It's a drug-o-rama.

1. Anti-inflammatory medication to reduce the swelling and pressure on the spinal cord. It also contributes to relieving some pain.
2. Pain medication for breakthrough pain. Maybe two kinds.
3. Tummy soother, especially if your anti-inflammatory drug is a steroid. Maybe two.
4. Muscle relaxant.
5. Sedative (for the dog, not you—ask your own doctor for one for yourself).

Use the Crate Rest Medications worksheet on page 127 to assist in discussing medications with your veterinarian and to ensure your dog has a separate drug for each need. Your veterinarian may prescribe additional medications for other needs or make substitutions.

More About the Five Types of Medication

1. The **anti-inflammatory** drug is the most important. This drug is your star player—the medication that will actually reduce the spinal cord's swelling and pressure, allowing it to heal. There are two types of anti-inflammatories: steroids and NSAIDs.
    - A common steroid used for IVDD is prednisone. Prednisone is stronger and cheaper than an NSAID, but it has more side effects. Common side effects are increased hunger or thirst (which leads to a need to urinate more frequently), gastrointestinal irritation, and bleeding ulcers. Also, a dog taking prednisone must be weaned off it to avoid damage to other organs. And (yes, there is more), a dog taking a steroid cannot take an NSAID without a four- to seven-day break, called a washout period, between them.
    - Common NSAIDs are rimadyl, metacam, and deramaxx, although there are others. NSAID stands for Non-Steroidal Anti-Inflammatory Drugs. NSAIDs are not without their own risks and side effects.
2. Pain medication for **breakthrough pain**. Most IVDD dogs also need a second pain reliever, especially if the anti-inflammatory is given only once a day.
    - Tramadol is very common for breakthrough pain. Be sure to ask your veterinarian how often you can give this drug to your dog. Ask for a schedule to give it (not just "as needed." It is much harder to get rid of pain once it starts, so you want to prevent it in the first place). Ask how much leeway you have to give extra. Tramadol is extremely bitter, so you'll need a really good, smelly, strong-tasting treat to give it, like liverwurst sausage. Also, Tramadol can have slight sedating effects.
    - Gabapentin (Neurontin) is another drug commonly used for breakthrough pain in dogs. Many vets believe that it is especially helpful for neurologically related pain. It may also have sedating effects.

Your dog should not be in pain during crate rest. Pain should be under control within one hour of receiving the first pain medication. After that, you should be able to manage pain with your prescribed dosage and frequency. If your dog is still experiencing pain, ask your veterinarian to adjust dosages or frequencies, especially with the breakthrough pain medications.

3. **Tummy soother**. If your veterinarian prescribed prednisone to reduce the inflammation of your dog's IVDD rupture or bulge, don't wait for bloody poop and loss of appetite. Go ahead and get your dog on some Pepcid AC, available over the counter. Ask your veterinarian for the appropriate dose for your dog's weight. The typical dachshund will take 5 mg twice a day. Many vets also recommend a tummy soother for dogs on NSAIDs. Your vet may give you a different soother, or the generic for Pepcid, famotidine. For extra protection against tummy upset, give your anti-inflammatory with food.

4. **Muscle relaxant**. Many dogs will involuntarily tighten other muscles to try to alleviate the pain in their backs. This can cause painful spasms in those muscles. Methocarbamol is commonly prescribed during IVDD episodes to help those muscles relax. Most muscle relaxers have sedating effects.

5. **Sedative**. Some dogs are very agitated by being in the crate. If you did not crate train your dog before the need for IVDD crate rest, she will not understand why she is in there now. This is upsetting for everyone. Just at the time when she is most upset, and in pain, and you want to comfort her, she feels she is banished to the crate, alone. Everyone feels betrayed and horrible. But more importantly, agitation prevents your dog from keeping still, which is absolutely necessary for the spinal cord to heal. A little chemical help can really make a difference. Your dog may get enough sedation from the breakthrough pain relief and muscle relaxer, but if she doesn't, request a calming drug like Alprazolam, otherwise known as "doggie Xanax."

Backup Plan. If you are not able to control your dog's pain at a time when your veterinarian's office is closed, you will need a backup plan. Ask your vet now what you should do, so you can save an expensive trip to the emergency clinic.

Setting Up Your Taj Ma-Crate

You want to set up the best crate ever, right? Let's not call it crate rest, let's call it Taj Ma-Crate Rest. To keep your dachshund as happy as possible during these eight weeks of confinement, your crate has to be awesome. Here's how to do it.

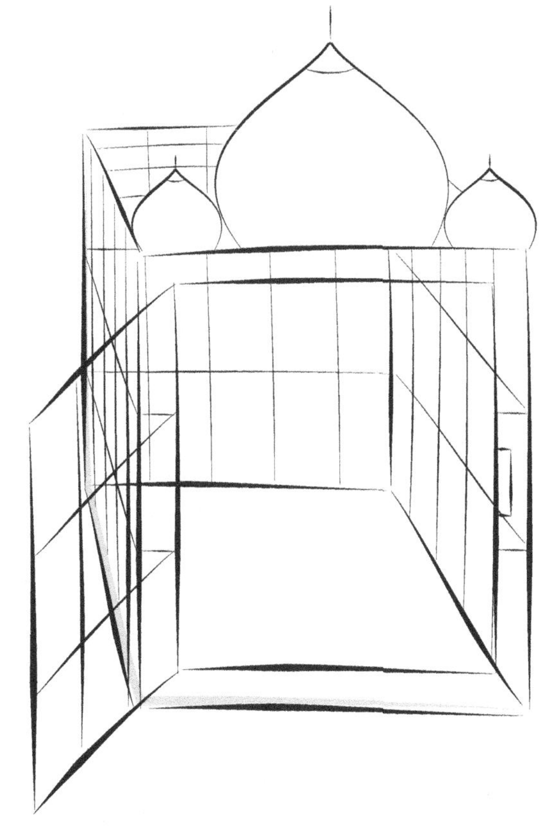

Where Should the Crate Be?

You may need to experiment with the best place to put the crate, depending on your dog. First, try putting the crate in the middle of things. You want your dog to feel as normal as possible, not separated from her family and pack. She's in pain! She doesn't feel good. She's druggy. You don't want to add to her distress and confusion by making her feel banished. Keeping her near you will help reduce agitation and unnecessary movement.

If you spend most of your time in the living room, that's where the crate should be. If you watch TV in the bedroom, put her crate next to your bed. If she is used to sleeping with you, put the crate on a chair next to the bed so she is on the same level. If she has a favorite napping spot and you can put the crate over that place, do it. Many doxies like to be near the heating vent. If yours is a vent hog, set the crate next to the vent.

Some people put the crate on a little wagon so they can wheel their lovebug from room to room as they move, like a little queen on her litter, carried by the servants. (Which, let's be honest, is how she views you anyway.)

Some dogs, though, need more isolation to calm down. If you dog just cannot settle, try putting her in a different room that offers more quiet. Experiment with putting the crate in one room during the day and another room at night. The best placement of the crate may take a few days of trial and error, and it may shift over the eight weeks.

What Goes in the Crate?

Put in a comfy cushion and a blanket. If she has a favorite soft toy, put that in. You want her to be warm and snug. You want her to feel safe. Consider buying several inexpensive cotton bathmats covered with a layer of fleece to wick away moisture. You can fold them in half for a soft but tidy surface, and they wash easily.

Some dogs feel better if you drape a blanket over the crate and make it into a little cave.

The Entertainment Schedule

The more you can keep her brain occupied in the crate, the less she will fuss. Since she probably doesn't read trashy magazines or watch movies, like we do when we are sick, we need to give her the dachshund equivalent—the Stuffed Kong.[9]

Crate Rest Shopping List

- Crate (duh)
- Crate cushions (at least two)
- Cheap bathmats
- Fleece blankets
- Soft blankies for burrowing
- Pill splitter
- Small, heavy, tip-resistant water dish
- Kongs (at least three)

[9] If your dog has a cervical disc problem, you may not want to use Kongs or chews, since both involve neck movement. Talk to your veterinarian.

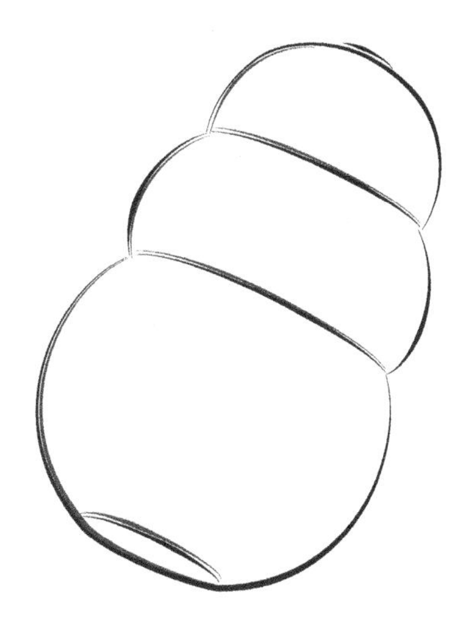

A Stuffed Kong will take you a long way. Get yourself three or four Kongs, those bulbous, hollow pyramid toys that you can get at any pet supply store. Then head to the grocery to buy any combination of the following:

- Plain yogurt
- Canned pure pumpkin
- Cheese (either a hard cheese that will cut into small cubes or cream cheese)
- Peanut butter (ideally low-salt)
- Chicken baby food
- Liverwurst

Back at the Taj Ma-Kitchen, mix any combination of the above together. Maybe add some of your dog's regular food to the mix. Squish this unholy goop to fill the Kongs (or you can just poke it into the Kongs in layers). Make sure there's a nice, smooth surface across the Kong opening. Then freeze. (Freezing the Kong is not strictly necessary, but it does help the treat last longer.) Put the rest of your delicious ingredients in the refrigerator so they are handy for refills.

Give your dog a Stuffed Kong when you leave for work in the morning, and any other time she seems unhappy with the crate. Re-stuff and re-freeze the Kongs as she goes through them, so you have a neverending supply of Crate Entertainment. This is like buying your dachshund the super-deluxe cable TV package.

What About Food and Water?

This is the Taj Ma-Crate, after all, and it includes room service. Put the water in a small, shallow, heavy dish that isn't likely to get tipped over. A flat-bottomed ceramic bowl is ideal.

Depending on your frozen Kong mixture, you may want to replace regular meals with the Kong. You do not want weight gain during this process. Excess weight just makes everything else that much more difficult. Control the higher-calorie components if you can. Your main concern is to keep your dog as happy and calm as possible, without tummy upset. Experiment to see what works. You may need the really yummy stuff at first, before everyone gets used to the routine, but be able to taper off to the less rich stuff after a few days. Keeping the diet as simple as possible will help to ensure healthy (read: non-disastrous diarrhea) bowel movements.

Does My Little Darling Really Have to Stay in There Alone, All of the Time?

You'll hear a hundred different opinions on this, all of them passionate. This is mine: Your dog needs to stay in the crate the vast majority—99.9 percent—of the time. But we all need love, especially when we aren't feeling good or feeling scared. That goes for both of you. I think it is fine, and maybe even emotionally necessary, to take a dog out of the crate for daily snuggle time, especially if you are doing something like watching a movie and you can sit closely together safely. Use the utmost care, and acknowledge the risk. Never forget that a dog can do the unexpected in the blink of an eye, like dart at the sight of a squirrel out the window or the sound of footsteps on the front porch. This is a judgment call each of us must make on our own. Make your call wisely and objectively. And keep your hands on your dog at all times when she is out of the crate. Every second.

The Potty Schedule

Crate rest, you will recall, means keeping still. Keeping still means no walking. No walking means you carry your dog outside to go potty. You don't allow even one more step than absolutely necessary. Carry your dog from the crate to the door, carry your dog outside, carry your dog down the back steps and into the yard to that favorite potty spot. Hold your dog up into a good position, and make all the encouraging "go" sounds you know (or express, if you need to).

After your dog delivers the goods, go right back inside and put her right back into the crate. Do this for the entire eight weeks—even after your dog starts to feel better. Remember: *Eight* weeks.

Crate Rest Troubleshooting: You're All Set Up. Now What?

You've set up the most royally pampering Taj Ma-Crate situation anyone could dream of. You've actually considered freezing a Kong full of Merlot and climbing in there yourself. What could possibly go wrong?

Problem	Initial Thoughts	More Reflections
Not eating	Loss of appetite could be a sign of pain, or nausea from one of the meds. Talk to your veterinarian.	It is unlikely that your dog is on a hunger strike to protest being in the crate, but that is possible. If the veterinarian does not think appetite loss is pain-related or a side effect, tempt your dog with different food. Chicken baby food and liverwurst seem to be the trump cards for hunger strikes. If those aren't gobbled up, you're probably dealing with pain or nausea. Are you getting the Pepcid in?
Not drinking	As with food, refusal to drink can be a symptom of pain or nausea. Try putting a no-salt, no-onion broth in the bowl to encourage drinking. (You can make this easily by boiling a chicken thigh in water.) If your dog doesn't drink that, she probably has pain or nausea. Talk to your veterinarian.	Not drinking is especially concerning if your anti-inflammatory is prednisone. One of prednisone's classic side effects is increased thirst, so a dog on prednisone that refuses to drink should be seen by a veterinarian.
Wet blankets	Figure out whether "wet" means water or urine. See below.	
Water spilling on blankets	Use a different bowl. You want a bowl that is shallow enough so that your dog doesn't have to move too much to get to the water, but that's solid enough that it won't tip over. A small, heavy, ceramic bowl is less likely to tip and wet the bedding.	You can also try one of those pet rodent waterers to attach to the side of the crate.
Leaking urine	You're probably dealing with one of two bladder problems: 1. Your dog may not actually have the ability to pee independently after all, leading to her bladder overflowing. You will need to express the bladder until that ability comes back. Quick test: If your dog squats or "postures" to pee when you go outside, she can probably control the bladder. 2. If your dog can control the bladder, but the bedding has urine on it, you need to give your dog the chance to pee more often. This is especially likely if you are using prednisone. You will need to go outside more frequently (every two to three hours until the prednisone is weaned off) or arrange for someone to take your dog out while you are at work.	Many people who come to me for coaching were told by their vets that their dog could urinate on her own when the bladder was actually just overflowing. Their dog's bladder actually did need to be expressed.

Problem	Initial Thoughts	More Reflections
Pain not controlled	The typical signals of IVDD pain are shaking, crying, tight tummy muscles, arched back, refusal to move, and refusal to eat. But look for signs that contradict each other. Is she moving around in the crate, but also crying? Is she eating, but also shaking? If the back is arched and the tummy is tight, your dog likely needs more pain relief. If she isn't moving around at all, she probably has pain. But if the only signals of pain you are seeing are crying or shaking, that is probably just unhappiness with the status quo. Also, you know your dog. If she normally shakes when she just wants something, shaking may not be a reliable sign of pain. Be strong, and be aware.	This is a difficult one, as the signals of pain can look very much like "I want out of here! I don't care how nice you think you made it! I want to be with you."
Restless, but not in pain	Ask your veterinarian about a sedative. Use your judgment. If she is moving around so much that you fear the crate rest isn't really rest at all, you need to either calm her or get her out of the crate to lie quietly with you. This, of course, should be a last resort. But some dogs just can't be still enough to get the "rest" part of crate rest. If you go this route, use extreme care so that she does not walk away or jump down from your bed or couch. If you get up, even for a second, put her back in the crate until you sit back down again. She should never be outside of the crate unless she is right by you with your hands on her body. You might also consider whether you need to move the crate to an isolated area. A Dog Appeasing Pheromone (DAP) product might also help keep her calmer.	Pain is an important signal from the body that something is amiss. If your dog is jumping around in the crate like nothing is wrong, ask your veterinarian about decreasing the breakthrough pain medication (not the anti-inflammatory). You don't want her to be in pain, but a little discomfort may discourage movement.
Not pooping	Is she eating? If she is eating, there should be pooping (simple gastrointestinal math). If nothing is going in, of course nothing is going to come out. Some dogs are so discombobulated by all the stress and pain and vet visits and change, they just don't poop for a couple of days, and that is probably okay. Maybe she won't poop the first day of crate rest, or even the second, but she definitely should poop by the third. If she is eating, but hasn't pooped by the third day, help her out. Lube up a Q-tip and twirl it around just inside the opening of her rectum.	If your dog isn't eating because she is in pain, that is a different situation. Poop will not come out, because there is no poop. See "Not eating" above.

Problem	Initial Thoughts	More Reflections
Blood in poop, but at least it is solid	This is almost certainly due to the anti-inflammatory drug or stress. Give Pepcid AC twice a day. If it doesn't resolve in a couple of days, call your veterinarian.	Consider a bland diet of chicken, rice, and plain yogurt.
Having diarrhea, and I just can't take any more of this!	Take deep breaths (but not in the room with the diarrhea). Diarrhea during crate rest is a nightmare. We are going to knock that out—never fear. First, notify your veterinarian and be prepared to answer questions about color and quality. If there is blood in the diarrhea, they may prescribe metronidazole (Flagyl) for colitis. Unless otherwise advised by your veterinarian, try withholding food for about 12 hours, but give your dog plain, salt-free broth to make sure she doesn't get dehydrated. After that, offer a very bland food, like boiled plain chicken and rice, for two days, with the Pepcid AC. Gradually return to a more normal diet.	For your frozen Kongs, stuff the Kong with chicken and rice and yogurt. Put this through the food processor to make your Soon-To-Be-Famous Chicken Goo. This bland mixture is friendlier to the upset tummy.
Weird muscle spasms!	Some IVDD dogs have weird muscle spasms or head bobs. In most cases, it is not something to be alarmed about.	If the spasms seem to be painful, especially if you are otherwise unable to control pain or if they are affecting the front legs, they could be a symptom of myelomalacia. Only a small number of dogs with IVDD develop this condition, but you need to be prepared to deal with it swiftly and with compassion if that happens. See the Glossary and page 57 for more information. Contact your veterinarian immediately if you suspect myelomalacia.
Arched back	An arched back is a sign of pain. The site of injury might be tender to the touch. Talk to your veterinarian about the medication schedule, especially the breakthrough pain medication. Another potential culprit is muscle spasms. Ask your veterinarian about a muscle relaxant.	Ask your veterinarian if there are any exercises you can do at this point that will not risk the spinal cord's healing process. For example, stretching to reach for a treat out of your hand can help assuage the tense muscles. Gentle massage may also help relieve the spasms.

Finding Your Crate Rest Groove

You're all set up, and you're ready to deal with any problems that come along during the eight weeks of crate rest. Now, what will this actually be like?

A typical day of crate rest looks something like this:

- 7 a.m. Carry your dachshund outside to potty; give breakfast with morning anti-inflammatory, breakthrough pain pill, muscle relaxant, and Pepcid AC.
- 8 a.m. As you leave for work, get a frozen Kong out of the freezer and put it in the crate. Give her sedative in a treat.
- 12 p.m. If your dog is having trouble with pain management (especially at first), have someone go over to give her a breakthrough pain pill in a treat, and perhaps another Kong. If she's on prednisone, she will need to pee as well.[10]
- 5:30 p.m. Home from work, carry outside to potty, dinner time, snuggles. Re-stuff her morning Kong and put in freezer. Breakthrough pain pill if needed.
- 7 p.m. Evening anti-inflammatory, muscle relaxant, and Pepcid AC. TV and snuggle time.
- 11 p.m. Last carry outside for potty. Breakthrough pain pill and sedative in a treat. Night-night Kong.

Of course, specific medication times will vary by prescription, but this schedule should give you an idea of how to balance it.

At the end of the first week, everyone will have settled into a routine with much less fussing and dramatics. Pain should be reliably under control, and the need for the breakthrough pain meds should decrease dramatically. Breakthrough pain meds should become less and less necessary over the course of the eight weeks.

For Paralyzed Dogs

If your dog was paralyzed, you probably will not see any gains in functionality for a while. As you progress through the eight weeks, one of three things will happen:

1. Your dog's pain symptoms will lessen, and she will start to show return of functionality—trying to stand up, posturing to pee, taking wobbly steps.

[10] Dogs on prednisone will need to empty their bladders much more often than dogs on other anti-inflammatories. Prednisone increases thirst, so these dogs drink much more and need to be expressed several times during the day.

2. Your dog's pain symptoms will lessen, but she will not show signs of regaining functionality.

3. Highly unlikely: Your dog's pain will suddenly get much worse.[11]

In either of the first two situations, your response needs to be exactly the same (except for the celebrating): Continue the eight weeks of crate rest to the bitter, bitter end.

What Else Can I Do? Add-on Therapies for Crate Rest

In the section "Do We Need More Rehab?" on page 68, we summarize a lot of different therapies that can be extremely effective in restoring function. But you may be thinking, "What else can I do now?" The answer is "Hold on, Nellie!"

During crate rest, there is very little else you can do. You do not want to start any kind of movement-based physical therapies because those movements interfere with the "rest" part of crate rest. The last thing you need is anything that gets in the way of healing the spinal cord. Movement gets in the way of healing. Your focus really needs to be on the rest and the meds. These help the inflammation subside and allow the spinal cord to heal.

> **Hold on, Nellie!**
>
> Crate rest is not the time for action. Crate rest is the time for patience and watchfulness and compassion and love...
>
> ...and drugs.

I know—this is difficult for you Type A's out there, who want to take a lot of action and do everything you can do. But crate rest is not the time for action. Crate rest is the time for patience and watchfulness and compassion and love.

Limit any add-on therapies you choose during crate rest to things that fit two criteria:

1. They do not involve movement.

2. They do involve fighting inflammation.

The add-on therapies that fit these criteria best are laser light and acupuncture.[12]

Laser Light Therapy.[13] More and more, regular veterinarian offices are investing in cold lasers for general anti-inflammatory and pain management uses. These are not the lasers used for laser surgery. Please discuss

---

[11] See a veterinarian immediately and specifically ask about myelomalacia.

[12] Hyperbaric oxygen therapy (HBOT) is beginning to receive some positive attention for reducing inflammation, but this therapy is in the early stages of experimentation and very difficult to find for dogs.

[13] Note that laser light therapy (or cold laser) is completely different from the lasers used for laser surgery.

with your veterinarian whether laser makes sense for your situation. Some veterinarians question the effectiveness of laser light for spinal inflammation, as the light does not penetrate the vertebrae. If your veterinarian does not have a cold laser, you can always use a different veterinarian just for that therapy. Ask your regular veterinarian to make a recommendation and send your records there.

Transportation Tip

When transporting your dog to therapy, just put the whole crate, dog and all, in the car. Don't add any more transitions in and out of the crate than you have to. Each transition is another movement.

Acupuncture. Make sure your acupuncturist is extremely careful to minimize moving your dachshund around during the session. No flipping her over, for example. Find a position and stick with it.

Reminders

- Crate rest is a marathon, not a sprint.
- It's an eight-week marathon, and there is no way to improve your time.
- You have two jobs: providing space and time to heal, and controlling pain.
- At some point, your dog will start to feel better, either because the pain has subsided or because function is returning, or both. Be strong until the eight weeks are over.
- You can do this.

From the Desk of Dr. Christman

Ancillary therapy is super important for the healing process. I am a huge fan of complementary medicine such as acupuncture. Be consistent with the sessions, and they can truly help your furbaby recover safely and more quickly. If you can find a facility that offers physical therapy, and underwater treadmill exercises after crate rest is complete, you will be well on your way to regaining ambulation.

—Adam Christman, DVM, MBA

The Big M

Let's talk about myelomalacia (even though we really don't want to).

The symptoms of myelomalacia are extreme distress (possibly acting feverish) with an anxious expression that has been described as "knowing they are going to die." Some dogs will have muscle spasms in the front legs as the condition moves upward. At an advanced stage of myelomalacia (if it is allowed to progress to that point), the dog will have difficulty breathing and eventually suffocate when it reaches the nerves that control the lungs. This process, left unchecked, will take two to three days. Myelomalacia is very painful and terrifying for a dog. We do not have a complete understanding of what causes it to happen.

Myelomalacia is fairly uncommon in dogs with IVDD ruptures—different sources estimate it will occur in three to 10 percent of all spinal cord injuries (that is, not just those related to IVDD). But it deserves a mention because of its horrific nature. It usually starts within 72 hours of the original injury, so if you are beyond that point, you can probably cross it off your list of worries.

If you suspect myelomalacia, you must get help from a veterinarian. Immediately. Do not wait. Even if that means an emergency veterinarian. Do it. If your dog has progressive myelomalacia, the kind thing to do is to put her to sleep. Myelomalacia is not a pretty death. If your veterinarian gives you this diagnosis, or a strong belief in one, the loving act is to let her go before she endures any further suffering.

i can't do surgery or crate rest. i just can't.

Well, let's be very honest then. That leaves you with just four other real choices.

1. Return to breeder
2. Find a new home
3. Rescue
4. Euthanasia

Only you can make the right decision—for your dog, for your family, for yourself. What I hope to do for you is to give you some things to think about as you decide. I hope to make you feel that you have a friend standing by you, not judging the direction you take, but being completely honest about your options and encouraging you to consider all the ramifications of each one. None of the directions are easy.

The Four Non-Treatment Options

1. Returning a dog to the breeder

If you purchased your dachshund from a breeder, check with them about what they want you to do with your dog as an alternative to euthanasia. Some breeders will want you to return the dog. If your breeder does want this, ask whether they will provide medical care.

Another reason to at least call the breeder, even if you don't want to return your dachshund, is to notify them that they have IVDD in their breeding stock and ask them to stop breeding both parents. IVDD is an inherited condition, passed down from parent to puppy.

2. Finding a new home

I'm not going to say that finding a new home for a dachshund with IVDD—even a paralyzed one—is impossible. It isn't impossible, but it certainly isn't easy, and it definitely isn't fast. Finding a new home for any dog takes some time. In the meantime, you will have to manage your dog's pain. That means you have to start the crate rest and medications anyway.

There are a lot of dogs in the world that need homes, and there are only so many homes to go around—even for the young, healthy, purebred dogs. When you were looking for your dog, you probably didn't consider an adult dog with health issues. Most people don't.

There are not very many people out there looking to adopt a dog with acute health issues. Taking care of an IVDD dog, especially in the first couple of weeks, can be challenging and scary. It is something most people do for a dog they already love, not a dog they don't know.

And of course, there are a lot of jerks out there, and a lot of hoarders out there. You don't want your dog to go into a situation that is even worse than the one she is in now. But you can try.

The best places to try are Facebook communities like Dachshund Lovers, Doxie Posse, and Dachshunds Rock! These communities are full of people who really love the breed, and many are familiar with IVDD. If you are very, very lucky, you will find someone who has experience with the disease, has decided that they will always have at least one disabled dachshund in their home, and is in a position to help you at the time you need it. If you find one of those people, count your blessings. You hit the jackpot.

It is tempting to post your dog on Craigslist, your neighborhood yard sale site, or other sites like that. True, these sites get a lot of attention and exposure. But there is a downside. These sites are often patrolled by people looking for free dogs to use for nefarious purposes like laboratory experiments or dogfighting bait. These sites can also attract homes who cannot afford veterinary care. Be very wary of anyone who is quick to jump on a "free dog" ad, especially for a dog who is hurt. Something is very likely not right about that person. They may have bad things in mind, or they may be prone to take on more than they can handle. It's certainly possible they have good intentions, but I urge you to use extreme caution when rehoming a dog with IVDD.

You need to find someone who is qualified. Someone who knows what they are doing or is at least willing to learn. You also need someone who does not already have so much on their plate that they get in over their heads.

Whatever you do, make sure the person knows what they are getting into and is comfortable with the commitment they are making. Follow up with them later, and offer whatever financial assistance you can with their vet bills. Your responsibility isn't over.

And manage your dog's pain until you find that home.

3. Rescue

You may find a rescue group that will be able to take your dachshund. But don't count on it. Rescue groups are constantly short on space and money. An IVDD dog requires a special kind of space. Not every foster home will take an IVDD dog. Even if the rescue has foster space open, that space may not be able to handle IVDD. All those foster volunteers are regular people just like you, who love dachshunds and want to help them. That doesn't necessarily translate to unlimited capacity to help every dog who comes along.

Rescue groups that specialize in dachshunds usually contain people in their organizations who are very familiar with IVDD. Most dachshund rescues have a couple of volunteers (the vast majority of rescues are completely volunteer-run) who are their go-to people for any dogs with back issues.

These go-to people have limits. I know, because I am one of them. But even though I know the ins and outs of IVDD care like I know the butt swirls on my own dachshunds' rear ends, I can only handle so much on any given day. My agreement with myself and my family is that I will foster one IVDD dachshund at a time, in addition to the two of our own. All of these go-to people have such limits.

This doesn't mean that a rescue group can't help, however. A rescue is more likely to be able to support you with coaching and getting online exposure for your dog. When you contact a rescue, ask whether anyone in their group is available for you to talk to on the phone, or even to visit, to see how they care for their IVDD dachshunds. Ask for a bladder expression lesson. Ask if they can list the dog for you on their website as a guest post so that potential adopters can see her. Ask if you can join one of their adoption events with your dog. Offer to make a donation. The best way to interact with a rescue group is to make it clear that you aren't trying push your problem off onto them—that you want a partner to help your dog, not someone to just "make it go away" for you.

You can find dachshund rescue groups on AdoptAPet.com and Petfinder.com. Do your research to make sure the groups you contact are well-respected. A few Internet searches should give you some clues as to whether they are reputable or not.

4. Euthanasia

We've come to the E Word. The scary thing. The hard, heart-wrenching thing.

Euthanasia is a tool in the veterinarian's toolbox. It is something your vet can do for you. So it makes sense that a veterinarian would offer it, and not the other three non-treatment options, which are services they cannot perform for you. Your vet probably cannot find a rescue, or another home, or contact your breeder for you, but your veterinarian can offer euthanasia.

To a veterinarian, the three available services are surgery, medical management, and euthanasia. Some veterinarians do not even know about the possibilities of crate rest with medications, so if surgery is not possible, they see euthanasia as the only other humane choice.

The sight of a paraplegic dog is not very common in our world, so most people, and many veterinarians, also are not aware of the high quality of life possible for an IVDD paralyzed dog, if all treatment options are unsuccessful.

Our belief is that euthanasia is warranted only if all of the following apply to you:

- Your treatments did not restore function.
- You are not able to care for a down dog now that you know what that care entails.
- Your breeder (if you have one) will not accept the dog's return.
- You are unable to find a qualified adopter or a rescue to take the dog in.
- You feel that quality of life is substantially compromised, and your dog's spirit is broken.

Of course, you need to think about the medical prognosis, your dog, and her quality of life. You need consider the physical aspects of your home and your schedule.

Quality of life for a down dog can be just as happy as quality of life for a walking dog. All of my paraplegic dachshunds wrestle, play ball, eviscerate toys, chase (and sometimes catch!) squirrels, worship sun-puddles, and enjoy burrowing and cuddling just like any other dachshund. One of my paraplegic dachshunds had the cheeriest disposition of the whole pack, even at 16 years old, after 10 years of being "down."

Care for a down dog is not that much more demanding than care for a walking dog. It's a little different, sure. It takes a few extra minutes a day. And yes, there's a bit of occasional cleanup involved. A sense of humor helps.

You also need to think about your family. If you have children, you have to think about the lessons they will learn about how we care for the ones we love. You have to think about whether the whole family will pitch in.

This is not a simple decision, and it surely is not an easy one. The most you can ask of yourself is that you make it with an open mind and an open heart, knowing that you weighed all the possibilities and exhausted all your resources.

If you do decide that you must say goodbye, try to be strong enough to hold your dachshund as she crosses over, telling her that you love her and that you did your best. You want her to leave this Earth with the dignity she deserves.

What Not to Do

If you're reading this book, you're probably not likely to do any of these things. But I've seen all of these things, more than once, from people who thought they were making a reasonable choice at the time. A lot of people don't know how these systems work. Desperate people do desperate things. If you're considering any of the below, you need to know what will really happen.

1. Don't leave your dog outside of animal control

What happens when you leave a dog outside of your local, government-run animal control agency: She will probably be considered a stray and will be held in a kind of legal limbo for at least three days, without pain medication, in a loud, smelly, scary place. When the stray hold period is over, your dog will be put down by people who do not care about her, in what may or may not be humane conditions.

Of course, there is a small chance that the animal control agency has a relationship with a dachshund rescue that also has space and finances to handle an IVDD dog at that moment. This chance is slight.

You're better off just going in and asking them to put the dog to sleep for you, in your arms if possible. If you request it, it will happen right away.

2. Don't report your dog "stray" so animal control will pick it up

This is the second-worst thing you can do. Some people call animal control and say that they found a hurt dog, even though it is actually their own dog. In these cases, the dog is definitely held for at least three days until the legal stray hold period is over. Most animal control facilities do not have medical funding or staff for pain medications. When the stray hold period is over, your dog will be put down.

3. Don't hope that a veterinarian will take over

It seems like a promising trick to leave your dog on the veterinarian's office porch in the middle of the night, or to run into the lobby and leave her on the floor for a veterinarian to leap in and save the day. What will most likely happen is that the vet will call animal control. If your dog is lucky, the vet will give her pain medication while she is still at the office, but then she will go to animal control and endure three days or longer before being put down. The veterinarian might call a rescue group, if they have relationships with rescues. But that's a big might. Most vets do not have those relationships. And then there's another big might about whether the rescue group can handle an IVDD dog financially and space-wise at that point in time. This isn't a good bet for your dog.

4. Don't count on a Good Samaritan to come along

This is the absolute worst thing you can do. Please, please do not just put your dog outside and hope that "someone" does "something." A "someone" probably will not come along at all. If "someone" even sees your dog, most people who see strays do nothing. If "someone" does take action, they most likely will call animal control. Until then, your dog suffers. Badly. Horribly. After she gets to animal control, if she even makes it there, your dog suffers again.

You Are the One in Control

You are the one in control of this situation, and as painful as it might be, you are the one who has to act.

Whatever choice you make, your family will need to talk carefully and honestly with one another about why your choice was the best one for your dog and your family. You need to consider what messages everyone may take from the experience, whether or not those messages are intended. Talking about all of this with love and honesty is best for everyone. Even if it is hard in the short term, it will be worth it in the long run.

part three: we got through the base treatment! what now?

Way to go! You made it through the acute part. Celebrate for a minute, and congratulate yourself. You deserve it. Now, what's next?

What to Expect After Your Base Treatment

If you chose surgery	If you chose crate rest
• The surgery is behind you, and the surgeon says it's time to move on. • Some dogs come out of surgery with full abilities and do not need any additional treatment, but many need a little help to get them back into the swing of things or to adjust to their new limitations.	• Eight weeks have passed in the crate, and you're both ready for the next step. • Like someone coming out of prison or a drug rehab program, your dachshund will need to adjust gradually to regular life when she rejoins society–sort of like a halfway house. • She will need to adjust gradually to spending time outside the crate. Start with short periods outside the crate when you are home, increasing by 15-minute increments. Let her start to figure things out on her own.

You probably find yourself in one of the four following situations—or at least, something pretty close to it.

1. YIPPEE!
2. Thumbs up!
3. Boo.
4. Dammit!

YIPPEE!

Everything is back to normal. Your dog can walk and run, pee and poop on purpose (or never lost these abilities in the first place), and do everything else!

- You can get back to normal life, with a few extra precautions to prevent future IVDD flare-ups. See page 119.
- Build up to normal activity gradually.

Thumbs up!

Your dachshund can walk, but it's a bit wonky. Pee and poop control is pretty good. Maybe not perfect, but good.

- Try a bit of physical therapy, either DIY or with a professional if you can find one. See page 68.
- Think about whether you need any adjustments to your home. See page 99.
- Take things slowly and don't overdo it. Increase activity a little each day.

Boo.

Your dachshund is still paralyzed in the rear legs but has some response to pain stimulus. The legs move in some situations. Perhaps she can "spinal walk." She can't pee on her own, but she seems to know that you're helping her express. Poop comes out, of course, just not when and where you want it to.

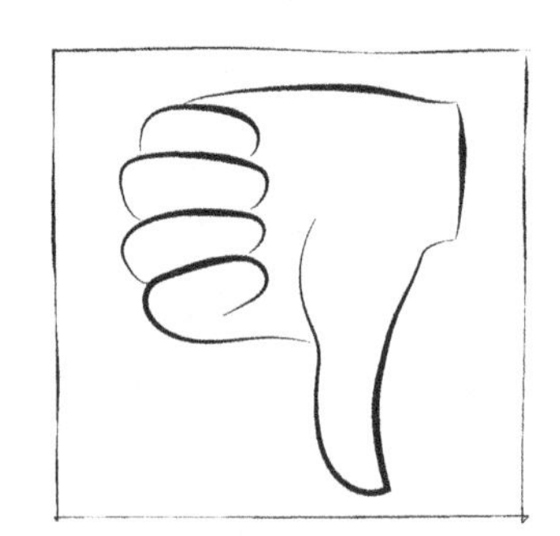

- Don't give up. Swim therapy can work wonders getting those signals to push through to the rear legs.
- In the meantime, resign yourself to regular bladder expression and dealing with the poop in whatever way you choose (Free to Be or OCD), at least for now. It's really not so bad.
- Sometimes dogs regain function after a few months. Sometimes they don't. The bigger questions are: Is she happy? Can you adjust?

Dammit!

Your dachshund is still paralyzed in her rear legs. There's very little, if any, sensation or movement in the legs. There's nothing going on bladder-wise at all. Poop does what poop does. You're in complete Nugget Land.

- Okay. That's really not what we wanted. And although the hope of walking again is not totally lost, it may be unlikely.
- Try swim therapy and other rehabilitation techniques.
- Look into wheelchair carts.
- I've seen dachshunds walk again after months of swim therapy, and I've seen them stall out right where they were after crate rest or surgery. There's no way to know your dog's true chances of walking again, or when.
- It may be time to accept a new reality. The new reality can be a very happy one. You're through the hardest part, after all.

What Is Spinal Walking?

Some dogs will move their legs in step-like movements, but will not seem able to coordinate the steps consciously. This strange, reflexive movement is called spinal walking or back walking. It is not the same as the actual ability to walk, but does that really matter? However your dog motors around is terrific, whether it is actual steps, spinal walking, or just scooting (with or without a special cart).

Some things are true no matter what.

No matter where you fall in the above situations, it's important to give your dog two opportunities in the first few weeks after completing base treatment:

1. Help her rebuild core strength in her chest and legs. After a few weeks of restricted activity, she may be a bit shaky and wobbly and weak, even if her function has returned. See page 69 for ways to do this.
2. Give her opportunities to struggle through what she needs to learn. The struggle has purpose. She is figuring things out—how to either get back up or how to cope with her new abilities. Maybe both at the same time. Plus, she wants to do things herself, just like a kid. If you see frustration, rather than just struggle, you can help. Otherwise, let her learn.

She's not a fragile flower—she's still a tough badger dog. She is still your dachshund who still likes all the dachshund things. You can both still be happy. It may be a slightly different happiness, but happiness nonetheless.

If function didn't come back, you're probably contemplating a full-on, two-year-old-on-a-crowded-airplane-style temper tantrum. And you probably want to say some very bad words. I get it. And I'm sorry about this. I would change it if I could, but I wasn't put in charge of this particular part of the universe.

Now is the time to begin rehab therapies that involve movement. Be gentle with her and with yourself. Some can be extremely effective.

the crazy ways function comes back

Do you remember the order that dogs lose function when a disc ruptures? They first lose proprioception (the ability to know where their feet are), then shallow pain, then deep pain.

Those abilities come back in the reverse order.

1. Deep pain will come back first. When you squeeze her toes, she will begin to pull back.
2. Then, shallow pain or sensation: She will begin to notice when you touch or brush her rear legs.
3. Then proprioception—she will start correcting her foot position instead of letting the toes knuckle under.

All of that *sounds* very neat and orderly, but the reality is often quite wonky as a dog recovers neurological function. Her legs may kick out spasmodically and without warning. She may pull her legs along one moment and take what looks like it might be a step the next. Function doesn't spring back to normal and fully recovered all of a sudden. It usually takes some madcap turns along the way.

Returning to Bladder Control: The Wacky Fire Hose

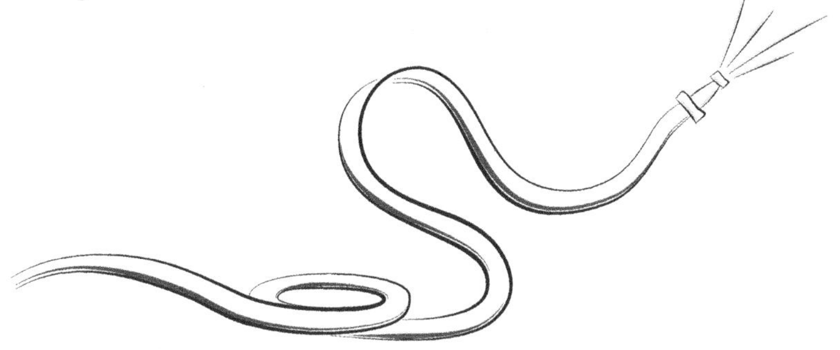

If your dog did not recover bladder control right away, you will hopefully see that start to come back during the first couple of weeks.

Remember, IVDD is freaky. And one of the ways it is really freaky is that healing can look like a backward step. Or sometimes a sideways, hip-hop kind of stumble.

Bladder recovery can be very strange indeed. The neural signals will start to go through to the nerves connecting the bladder, but not normally (at first). It may happen in fits and spurts (literally) in unpredictable patterns.

You may see what looks like a bad sign, but can actually be a good sign: Your dog may become incontinent for a while. Really incontinent, not overflowing. When you pick your dog up, urine may fly out as if from a firehose (especially for boys). Urine may leak even when he isn't full. Or he may be able to start to pee on his own (when you put him in position), but not finish. Or he may be able to finish peeing, but not start. Or he may go back and forth between all of these.

You can try a few different things to move this process along. Consider it one of your exercises. For example, if he starts peeing on his own but doesn't finish, give him a little help with some very gentle squeezes to see if he starts again. If he can't get started but can finish, start him very softly and see if he can finish with a little less pressure from you each time.

Even though this doesn't sound good, and it certainly isn't fun, it *is* progress. The wackiness may last a few days, but probably not longer than that. Buy some extra paper towels and floor cleaner, stock up on laundry detergent, and hold on tight. Keep in close contact with your veterinarian about any changes.

do we need more rehab?

Note: These tables do not recommend any specific therapies. Talk to your veterinarian or therapist about the treatments that interest you.

Therapies That Are Generally Safe During Base Treatment

Therapy	How It Works and Typical Goals	Where You're Likely to Find It	Can You Do It at Home?
Acupuncture	Encourages circulation and flow of energy.	Some regular vets, most holistic vets.	No
Laser (also known as cold laser)*	Reduces inflammation to promote healing. Note: Because the laser does not penetrate bone, and the spinal cord sits inside the vertebrae, some vets do not believe laser is effective for IVDD. It may, however, help with the muscles around the back.	Many regular veterinary clinics now have lasers. If yours does not, ask for a referral.	No
Brushing	Using a soft brush on the rear legs encourages nerves to rebuild their connections in the spinal cord. Some vets recommend doing this beginning right after surgery and during crate rest.	You can do this easily at home. A veterinarian rehab center can give you specific instructions if you are unsure.	Yes
Hyperbaric oxygen therapy (HBOT)*	Breathing inside a pressurized chamber, the dog absorbs oxygen, which reduces inflammation in damaged cells.	Difficult to find. Ask your veterinarian for a referral.	No
Herbal remedies and homeopathy	Supplements and techniques to stimulate healing and reduce inflammation.	Ask your veterinarian if they know of a holistic veterinarian who is competent in these practices.	Yes

* A DVM is probably required.

Therapies That Should Wait Until After Base Treatment Is Complete

Therapy	How It Works and Typical Goals	Where You're Likely to Find It	Can You Do It at Home?
Swim/aqua therapy/ hydrotherapy	A therapist supports your dachshund while she swims in warm water. The instinct to swim (and possibly the fear of water) forces neural signals through to the rear legs. Specific techniques encourage kicking the rear legs.	Veterinarian rehab center or aquatic therapist.	Yes
Standing in warm water	Helps dog regain balance by providing support to the body. The pressure of the water on the muscles also provides inherent benefits.	Veterinarian rehab center	Yes
Underwater treadmill	Especially useful for a dog already showing signs of walking on her own. Water provides body support while the treadmill encourages the dog to take steps and rebuild walking skills.	Veterinarian rehab center	No
Towel/sling walking	Sling provides body support while forward motion encourages rebuilding walking skills. Note: Also useful for just taking a paraplegic dachshund out for a spin if you do not have a cart!	Veterinarian rehab center	Yes
Chiropractic*	Realigns spine so neural signals can flow.	Laws and licenses vary widely by state. Some vets do it, some human chiros do it.	No
Massage	Increases circulation and flexibility. Relieves muscle tension. Relaxes dog to allow for healing.	Ask your veterinarian for a referral.	Yes
Other physical therapy exercises	Varied specific physical therapy activities to encourage a dog to relearn walking skills, e.g., passive range of motion, stretching, balancing on a soft beach ball, using a wobble board, and stepping over obstacles. Also useful for permanently disabled dachshunds to build strength or balance in front legs and chest.	Veterinarian rehab center	Some
Walking wheelchair cart	For dachshunds with spinal walking. Provides support to the body while the legs move.	Ask a rehab veterinarian or the cart manufacturer for assistance in measuring your dog for a walking cart.	Yes

* Chiropractic is very controversial for IVDD. Ensure you have a qualified chiropractor who is working with a qualified vet and that both of them are familiar with IVDD.

Finding a Physical Therapist or Rehabilitation Center

Veterinary physical therapy is a rapidly growing field. You may be surprised at how many resources are available in your area. While you can perform some physical therapy (PT) yourself, other treatments require equipment or expertise that is just not available to the typical dog owner.

Finding veterinary rehab can take a surprising amount of digging. Several professional organizations exist, and many of the schools have graduate lists. You will likely need to look in several places before finding anything or before finding something you like. A first step is to find the closest school of veterinary medicine to you. See if they have a physical therapy program, or call to ask for references.

To search the Internet for physical therapists in your area, use search terms like "veterinary rehabilitation center," "veterinary physical therapy," and "canine swim therapy" or "canine hydrotherapy." However, it seems that the all-powerful web-crawler algorithms are not yet skilled at finding veterinary physical therapists. I was surprised that several known rehab centers in my area did not come up with any of the above searches.

Performing PT at Home

If you plan to try PT yourself, the biggest thing to remember is to make it a fun and happy experience for your dachshund. Keep your home PT sessions short. Nothing you do at home should hurt. Get really special treats, or put some chicken baby food in a syringe and give your little one a tiny bead of it when she tries to do what you want. Be patient. Celebrate small victories.

part four: the paraplegic dachshund user manual

It may turn out that your dachshund never walks normally again. Not walking is not as straightforward as it sounds. It can take a lot of different forms:

- She may walk pretty normally, but with a bit of a wobble.
- She may walk as though her back end is drunk, occasionally falling over to one side.
- She may be able to run, but not walk. Some dachshunds, once they build up some speed, can get one rear leg under them, even though they can't take slower, deliberate steps.
- She may just scoot around, pulling her hindquarters behind her and developing some truly impressive chest muscles in the process, like an Olympic swimmer. Some people call this "The IVDD Shimmy."

IVDD is a strange disease, and it affects different dogs in a lot of different ways. It's difficult to predict how any individual dachshund may be affected. Neural signals get through in some ways, but not in others, with some weird effects.

In dachshunds with very severe ruptures, the muscles can eventually completely atrophy in the rear until the little rear legs just dangle uselessly. When they pull themselves around, their legs will be flat out behind them and their tails will remain on top of their bodies.

For most dogs, though, some muscle tone remains. Their legs may respond reflexively to some stimuli. When these dogs pull themselves around, they will use a sitting position, with the rear legs pointing forward as they drag themselves on their butts. Their tails tuck underneath.

In any case, she will still be a dachshund. She will still play, she will still chase balls and destroy stuffies, she will still beg for food, she will still get into trouble whenever the opportunity presents itself, and she will still do all the regular doggie things. Most dachshunds adjust very well to a paraplegic life, if that is how they end up.

The personality of the dog can be an important predictor. If your dachshund has the driving personality most dachshunds do, she will probably adjust just fine. If she never lets things get in her way, and if she is relentless about getting what she wants, she probably will not be distressed in the least by her new life. You will be much more bothered than she is by her dragging around, until you get used to her new way of motoring. But that's just another form of what my dear friend Michele calls "Homo Sapiens Bullshit." Try to let go of that—your dachshund would be baffled by your pity.

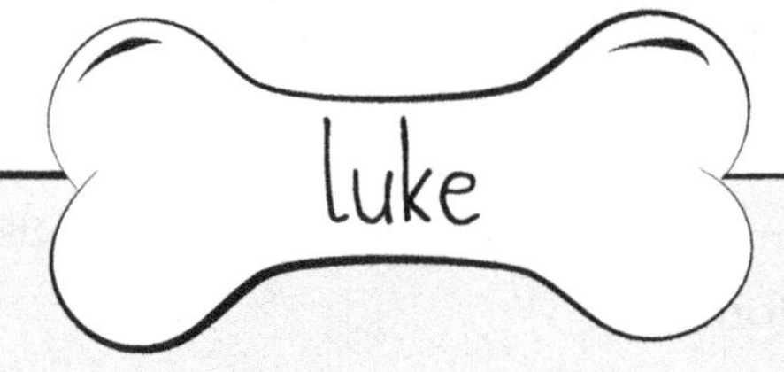

Luke

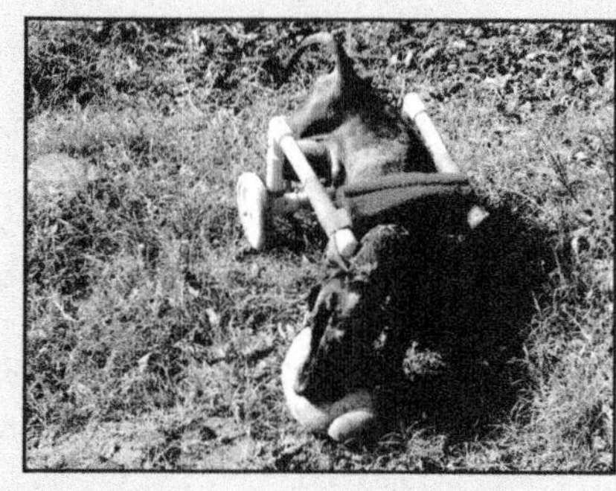

It must be admitted that Luke was kind of a jerk. Like the quarterback on many a small-town football team, he was good-looking and he knew it. Paralyzed at age five, his family took him to the vet when he showed signs of pain. The vet gave him a steroid shot and sent him home with no instructions about crate rest. That steroid shot made Luke feel great! Always a wild man, Luke leaped out of the car when they got home and went "down" in the driveway. His family surrendered him to rescue, who provided Luke with surgery.

Luke regained the ability to move his legs, but not the ability to walk right away. Like many dachshunds, he was protective of his territory. He would chase guests out of the house, scooting along to nip at the backs of their calves, but never hard enough that they would actually say anything beyond a startled screech. He knew his audience. After all, who is going to make a fuss about a nip from a small paraplegic dog?

We took Luke to swim therapy for months. One day, the therapist put him out of the pool and he ran to me! He had to go fast to get his momentum. In his cart, Luke could really fly. He liked the light PVC cart and was completely reckless in it, taking several spills on each outing. He was a daredevil. If there was a squirrel in sight, he was off like a shot.

Luke fostered with me for several months, until his best friend ever, Kim Hill, adopted him. Luke lived happily with Kim for several years until he passed away from causes unrelated to his IVDD.

—Kristin Leydig Bryant

joining the bladder club (aka finding the bladder)

Finding the bladder is the hardest part of learning to express it. But take heart—it isn't that difficult, and once you recognize the feel of a bladder between your fingers, you never forget it.

The first time you distinguish the bladder from all the other squishy stuff in a dog's abdomen, you will feel an unexpected surge of pride. Be prepared—you will probably whoop out loud. You will post online about your accomplishment, and it will earn a lot of "likes" (along with some baffled comments). You will wonder if there is a way to incorporate your new skill into your résumé.

Places We've Done It*

- Over the banister of a friend's deck (holding on tight).
- Out a parked car window.
- In many hotel room bathrooms.
- On the ramp of an interstate exit.
- In a formal gown and high heels, as the taxi beeps its horn to hurry up—it's New Year's Eve already.
- Outside a tent, camping, in the pitch-black darkness.

We can do it anywhere. it's easy.

So can you.

**Expressed a paralyzed dog bladder. Get your mind out of the gutter—this isn't that kind of book!*

How Do You Find It?

Horizontally, the bladder is located a couple of inches forward from where the rear legs attach to the torso. Vertically, the bladder is about halfway from the belly to the spine. It feels like a water balloon, and is about the size of a lime. Maybe a lemon, if your dog is a little larger or if the bladder is really full. An orange, if you've really let things go too long.

There's no other way to do this—you're just going to have to fumble around your dog's abdomen, feeling for the water balloon. You may want to ask a funny friend to join you, because this is going to be awkward, and you're already pretty freaked out, and you want someone who will make you laugh, even if you cry at the same time.

Take your dog outside and find a comfortable spot in the grass. Place your dog on the ground in as natural a standing position as she can manage. It's okay if her hindquarters don't support themselves. You can support her while you squeeze.

I think it's easier to find the bladder with one hand, but a lot of people start out using two hands. Begin squeezing around, trying different spots. Try to put the pad of your thumb into contact with the pad of your middle finger (or, if using two hands, try to touch your two middle fingers together). At first, you will feel nothing. You'll swear there is nothing in there but undefinable fleshiness. Keep groping. Keep feeling around. It may take a few tries. It *will* take a few tries.

Eventually, you will encounter the bladder, or you will see a little urine come out, or her legs may give a little twitch. That's it! You're in the right area. You found it!

From now on, when you meet other IVDD dog parents, you will shyly ask if you can try to find their dog's bladder. They will smile knowingly and give you permission. When you feel the new bladder, you will whisper to yourself, "There you are, my little beauty." The other owners will cheer, and they will ask if they can try to find your dog's bladder. You will hover over them, holding yourself back from giving advice. Your dog will roll her eyes.

You've joined the Bladder Club. Our secret handshake is built right in.

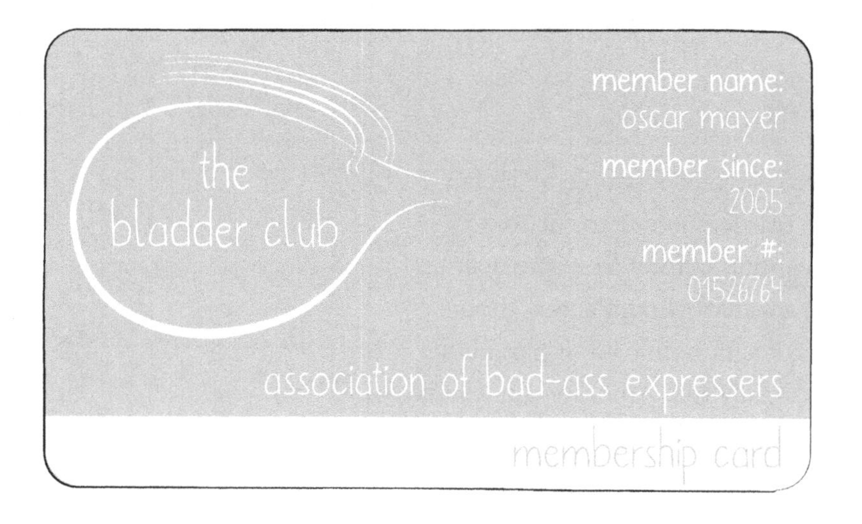

the urinary tract: what you need to know

From the Desk of Dr. Christman

The urinary tract is a dynamic process—constantly in motion. The basic functions of the urinary tract are to excrete toxic wastes from metabolic processes, regulate blood pressure and electrolyte balance, secrete hormones, and control the body's water balance and output in the form of urine.

The dog's urinary tract consists of a pair of kidneys, a pair of ureters, a bladder, and a urethra. The kidneys lie against the dog's abdominal wall. Kidneys are large filters—like the colander you keep in your kitchen. Their goal is to keep the good things in, while letting the bad things flow out through the remaining parts of the urinary tract. Each kidney has one ureter, a long tube that carries concentrated urine to the bladder.

The bladder is an incredibly resilient storage facility. Its walls are made up of a special type of tissue called transitional cell epithelium, which allows the bladder to stretch and expand as it fills and to relax and contract when it empties. The urethra carries the urine from the bladder to the outside of the body.

The bladder is a top concern for people who care for paraplegic dogs. A "normal" dog's bladder has plenty of nerve activity (also known as innervation). The bladder has two kinds of this activity: "fight or flight" (sympathetic innervation) and relaxation (parasympathetic innervation).

The sympathetic innervation dominates the filling phase of the bladder. As the bladder fills with urine from the kidneys, nerves stimulate the smooth muscle of bladder, resulting in contraction and forming that internal urethral sphincter. You and I experience that feeling every day with that "gotta go, gotta go" sensation. The hypogastric nerve, which exits the lumbar part of the spinal cord, supplies the sympathetic innervation.

Another nerve, the pelvic nerve, supplies the bladder with parasympathetic innervation. This nerve arises from lower spinal cord segments in the sacrum. The parasympathetic innervation signals the emptying phase in a series of coordinated steps. In the emptying phase, the bladder contracts and relaxes (creating that "Ahh, it feels so good to pee" feeling).

With a paraplegic dog, the emptying signals of innervation are not able to reach the dog's brain, and she needs help to empty her bladder. When you express your dog's bladder, you are supplying her bladder with a direct signal to void urine—the signal her brain cannot provide. You're also giving it a little bit of mechanical help by literally pushing the urine out.

—Adam Christman, DVM, MBA

in the food...

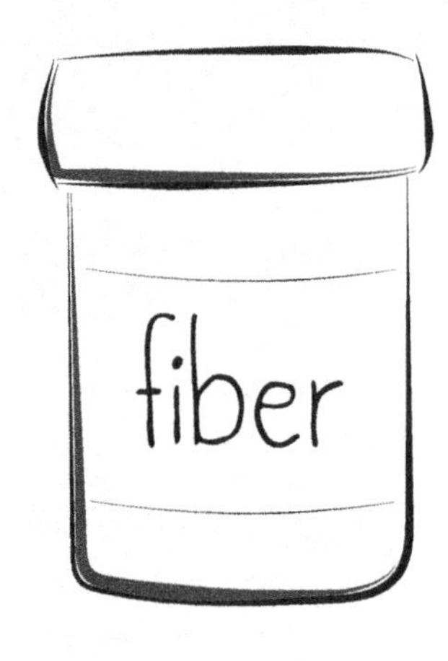

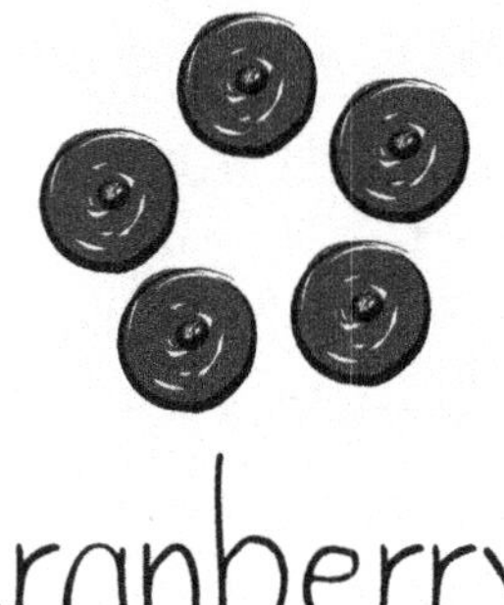

cranberry supplement

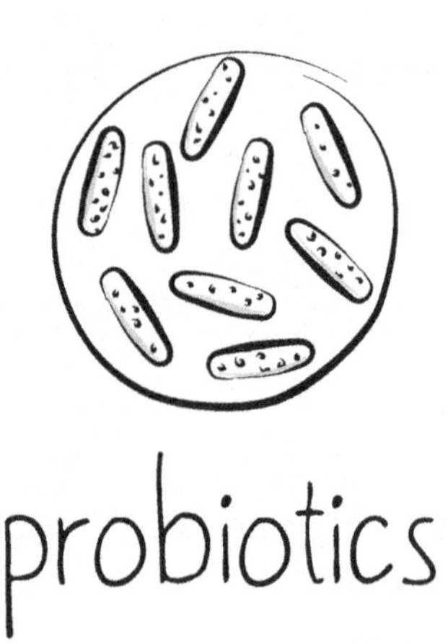

probiotics

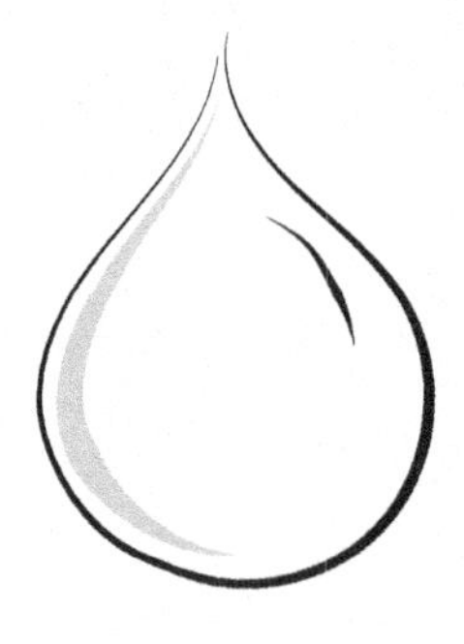

water

a daily schedule

Yes, I work a full-time job. No, that full-time job is not squeezing bladders.

7:00:00 – 7:00:20 a.m.

Squeeze bladder. (Yes, it takes less than one minute.)

7:15 a.m.

Breakfast with fiber, cranberry supplement, probiotics, and water.

Lunch

Squeeze bladder if you're home. Otherwise, skip.

5:30:00 – 5:30:20 p.m.

Squeeze bladder.

6:00 p.m.

Dinner with fiber, cranberry supplement, probiotics, and water.

Right before bed

Squeeze bladder.

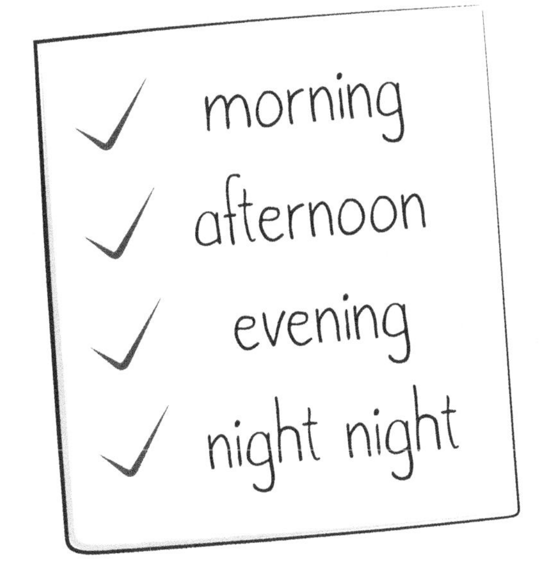

Why the Fiber, Cranberry Supplement, and Water With the Food?

The fiber supplement is to benefit you. No, I don't mean that you take it—you still give it to your dog. But you are the one that reaps the benefit. (Of course, if you want to take a fiber supplement, that is your business. But that's not the subject of this book.) Fiber makes for a nice, firm doggie poop that is much more pleasant to deal with. Fiber can be something as simple as a little canned pumpkin, or a psyllium husk supplement. We will talk more about this in the "Poops You Can Be Proud of" section on page 93.

The cranberry supplement, probiotics, and water are for them. A less active or older dog may not go over to the water bowl on her own until she is very thirsty, and then she will drink a large amount all at once. Drinking a large amount creates a higher likelihood of a suddenly full bladder. If you add a couple of tablespoons of water on the food—no biggie—you keep a more even supply of fluids running through her. The cranberry supplement and probiotics may help the bladder create an unfriendly home for bacteria.

order of operations

1. squeeze

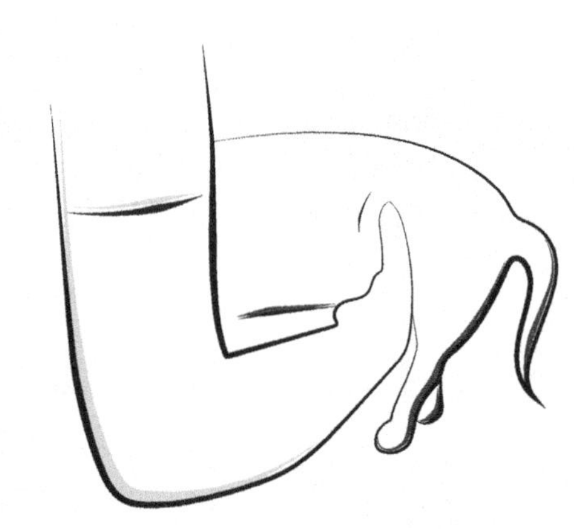

2. feed

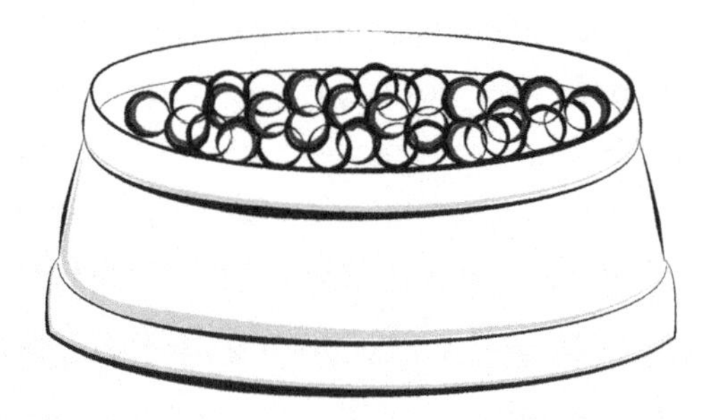

Squeeze, Then Feed

Did you notice that I squeeze the bladder before my dachshunds' meals, not after? Two reasons:

1. Just like we do, dogs need to "go" first thing in the morning. So, don't delay. Get right on that.
2. It is easier to express the bladder when the tummy is empty, especially when you are learning. (One less thing to get in your way.)

Easy peasy.

Timing the Bladder Expressions

From the Desk of Dr. Christman

It is important to think of the physiology of your dog's urinary needs. If my Cosmo is having an active, playful day, swimming in the pool or shimmying around playing, he's going to get thirsty. Especially on hot days, I know that he will drink more water to replenish lost moisture and electrolytes. So I also know that I will need to express his bladder a little earlier, and a little more often, on those days, because his bladder will fill up more quickly. If it is a cold and rainy day, you can bet Cosmo will be burrowed under a blanket in the house. I will not have to express his bladder more than three times on a day like that.

I tell my clients to express their paraplegic dog's bladder at least three times a day, or about every eight hours. First thing in the morning, an after-work squeeze, and one more before bedtime usually works for Cosmo, unless, of course, I know that he has had a thirstier day for some reason. On those days, the gap of time between expressions needs to be shorter, and I plan accordingly.

Regardless, you should have plenty of time for a normal quality of life yourself while attending fully to your dog's needs. A paraplegic dog doesn't need to urinate any more often than a dog who can "go" on their own.

—Adam Christman, DVM, MBA

the carry

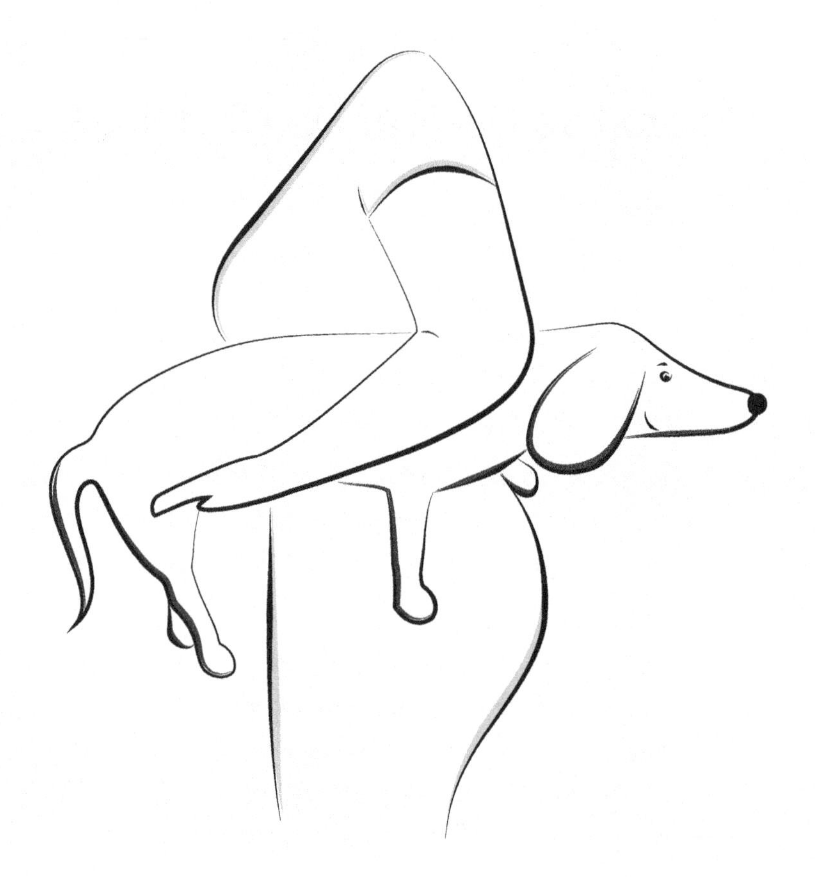

squeezing a girl

Now that you know how to find the bladder, and how often you need to express it, let's refine your technique based on the sex of your dog.

The Carry

When I'm getting ready to squeeze one of my girls, I pick her up and rest her on my forearm like a football, with her tail facing forward. My hand cradles her abdomen to keep her stable. As I walk, she is looking backward from under my arm, with her body against my hip.

Both girls find this position strangely comfortable, so much so that I sometimes forget and carry them this way even if we are not on the way to the bathroom. This can startle guests. If my husband encountered me en route with Tabby in this position, he often quipped something about "the business end of the Princess." Sometimes I responded by pretending Tabby was a machine gun, with accompanying sound effects.

The Basic Squeeze

Once you've learned to find the bladder, you'll figure out which way to squeeze works best for your girl. I can express Paris best when I squeeze her bladder at a steep downward angle, away from her tail, while Tabby's bladder squeeze was very direct and horizontal, toward the tail. Some bladders require a sort of rocking motion. You may feel that you are squeezing one end of the bladder toward the other. There is no "right" way—except for the way that works for your dog.

> Tabby's nickname was The Princess, which gives a whole other interpretation of that old fairy tale. We now think of it as The Princess and the Pee.

Squeeze the bladder over and over until it is flat, using about the same amount of pressure as you do to get toothpaste out of the tube. For my dogs, that is usually three or four squeezes. Squeeze until the walls of the bladder rub against each other, and you can't feel any more liquid. That's the feel of an empty bladder.

expressing a girl

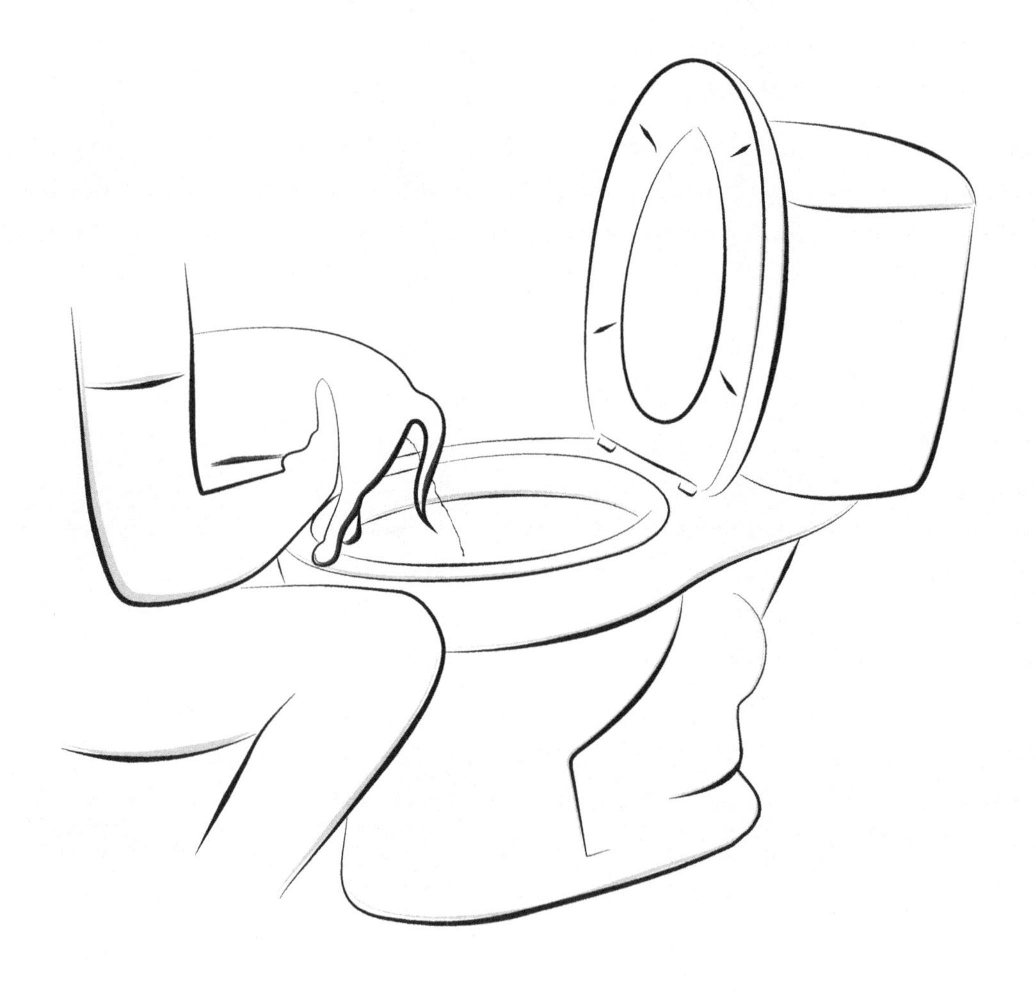

Advanced Maneuvers: Expressing a Girl Into the Toilet

It is extremely easy to express a girl over the toilet. Far easier and more convenient than trekking outside to do it. Just four steps:

1. Squat in front of the bowl (or drag in a chair).
2. Rest your dog on your thigh, with her bottom over the bowl.
3. Stabilize her body with your dominant arm. You may find it helpful to press down gently on her back with your non-dominant hand to trap the bladder and keep it from rolling around.
4. Use your dominant hand to find the bladder and squeeze until you feel the bladder flatten and empty.

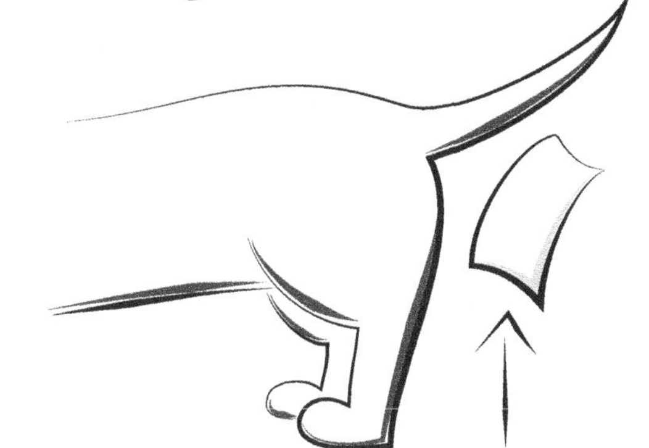

Usually, a little shake is enough post-squeeze cleanup. If you want to wipe, make sure you wipe upward so as not to spread UTI-causing bacteria from the rectum to her lady parts.

After a squeeze, give her a treat. Especially in the beginning, the treat will help her feel positive about this whole weird process.

squeezing a boy

When I brought my first paraplegic dachshund boy home, I thought expressing his bladder would be just like expressing my little girls'. Kind of direct.

No big deal, I thought. I've got this. How different can it be?

It's true, there are similarities, but there are some unexpected differences. The biggest difference is that you have to aim.

Difference 1: Aim

I'm a girl, so I've never had to aim my urine. And with Tabby, the first little paraplegic girl I took care of, who taught me almost everything I needed to know about this whole crazy IVDD thing, this was also true. I just held her bottom over the loo, found the water balloon of the bladder, squeezed, and out the pee came, in a nice, tidy, predictable arc. If you're taking little mister out into the yard and putting him in normal pee position to pee in the wild mountain air, no worries. But if you want to do it over the toilet, like I do (because I am lazy), you're going to have to learn to aim.

Difference 2: Orientation

Kind of like with humans: Girls sit. Boys stand. You have some choices on how to orient your little guy when you squeeze him. Will he be a vertical guy or a horizontal guy? An in-the-air guy or an on-the-ground guy?

Difference 3: The Crazy Straw

With girls, the urethra (the little tube from the bladder to the outside) is a nice straight pathway. With boys, that isn't the case at all. The urine has to make a hairpin turn before it comes out. It's not quite a crazy straw, but it sure can feel like it from the outside.

Boy Basics

When you're getting started learning to express a boy dog, I strongly recommend taking him out into the yard. He is used to going potty out there, and that's about the only thing about all this that will feel normal to him. You want him to be as relaxed as he can possibly be.

Stand your dachshund with all four feet on the ground in as natural position as you can, and feel for that water balloon. If his bladder is very full, it may be more toward his chest than you expect. If it's not full, it will not be very far from the base of his penis. Find it, and squeeze. Try some different motions: a milking motion, or squeezing from one end of the bladder to the other, in either direction. You'll have to find what works. (This is a highly personal matter, for sure.)

Squeeze the bladder over and over until it is flat, using about the same amount of pressure as you do to get toothpaste out of the tube. Squeeze until you can feel the walls of the bladder touch each other and you can't feel any more liquid. That's the feel of an empty bladder.

Once you have mastered this basic technique, you can move on to the more advanced "outside" techniques, or even the Master Squeezer technique over the toilet in the house.

What is common to every style is this: In all likelihood, your dog will look at you with his big brown eyes, and maybe even give you a kiss as you get started. He will know you are taking care of him.

He will probably bark for a treat afterward, so you'd better be prepared with that, too.

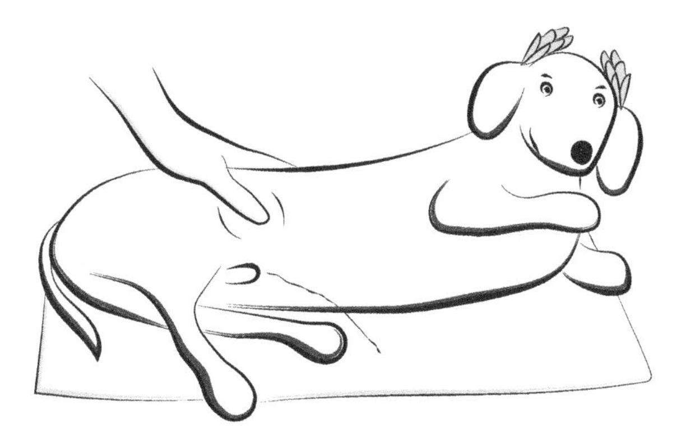

Style A: Roman Emperor

The dog lies on his side on a pee pad. You press on the bladder from one or both sides. This is the style often demonstrated by veterinarians and vet techs because the most common time a dog is expressed at the veterinarian is in conjunction with surgery, when the dog is unconscious and lying on his side. This style is less popular with dogs who are awake, but it can still be a useful way to learn.

Style B: Iron Man

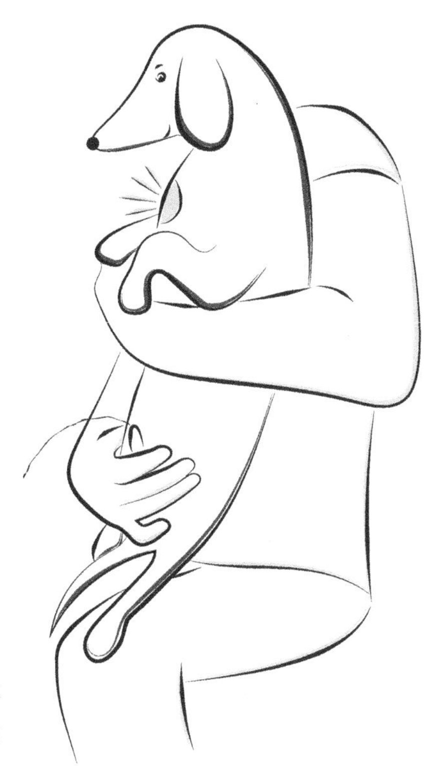

In this style,[14] you are standing, so it's good for people with bad knees or bad backs of their own. Hold your dog in a vertical position (as though he were standing up too). Support his bottom on your thigh, with your knee slightly bent. With your dominant hand, feel above the base of his penis for the bladder. Squeeze with your thumb and middle finger until the bladder is flat and empty. Tell your friends to step back, because things can get a bit unpredictable the first time or two.

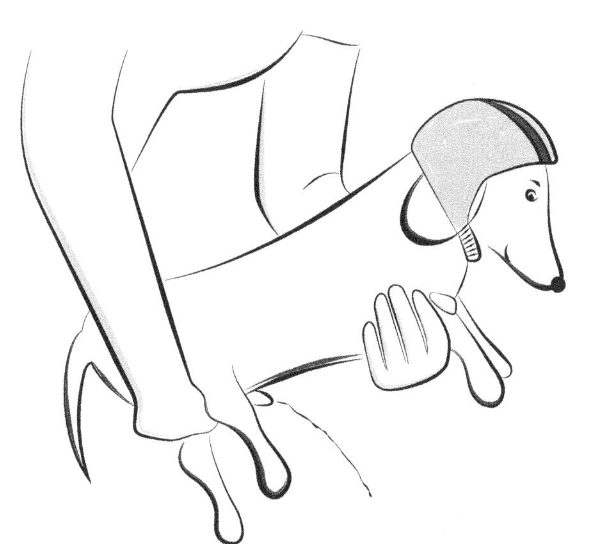

Style C: Quarterback

Very similar to the Iron Man, except that you hold the dog in a horizontal position. Balance him with your forearm and hand, and squeeze with your dominant hand until the bladder is flat and empty.[15]

---

[14] During crate rest or right after surgery, use only positions in which the back is horizontal.

[15] This is the style Dr. Christman uses in his YouTube videos.

master squeezer

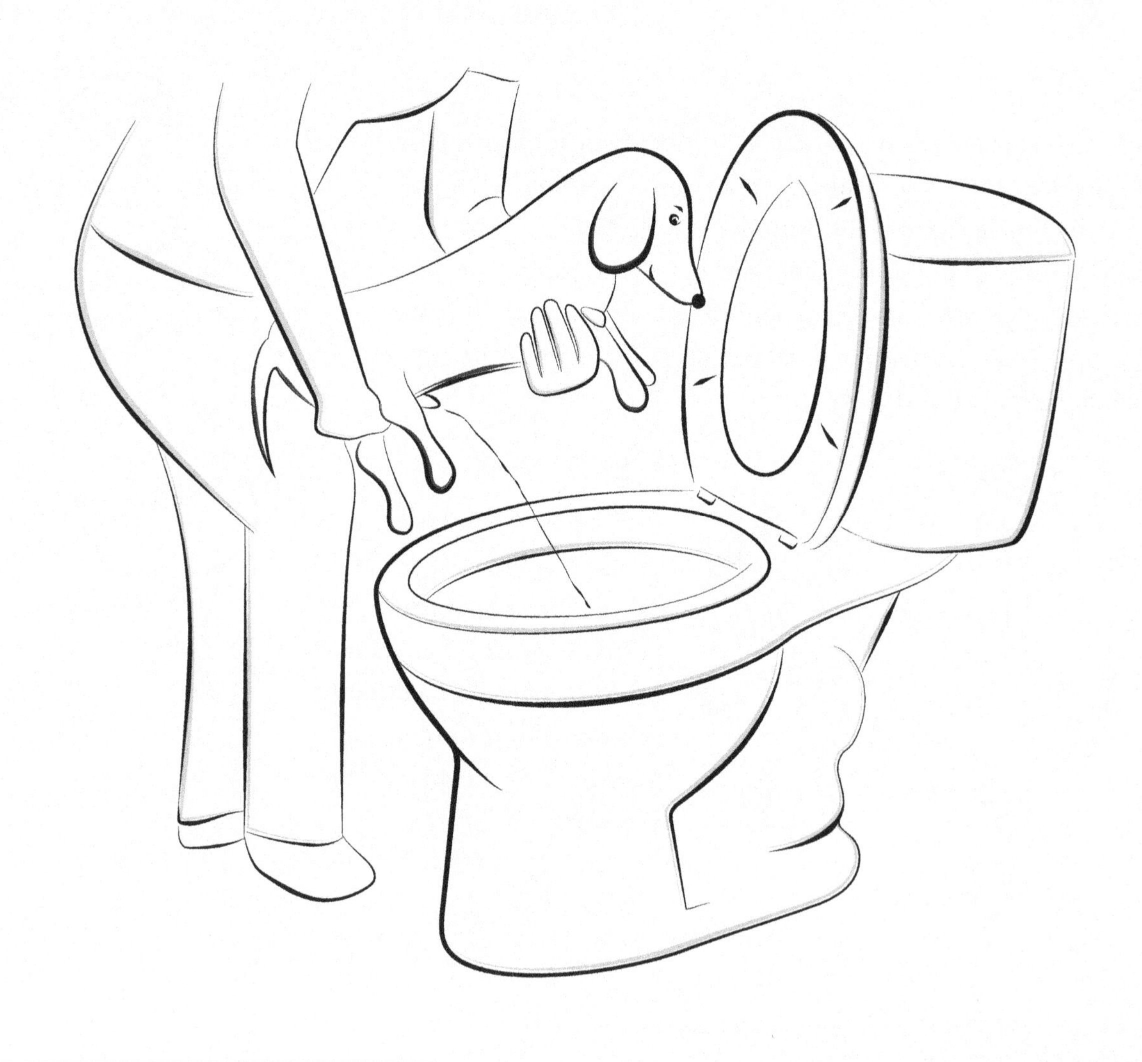

Style D: Master Squeezer

When you're feeling pretty confident, and you want to take your skills to the next level (as they say in corporate-speak), it is time to challenge yourself to the Master Squeezer—expressing your boy dog into the toilet. Go ahead and get out the disposable wipes; you're going to need them.

As with any (well-mannered) boy, raise the seat. Using the Quarterback as the base style, hold your boy over the toilet, getting him as close to the bowl as you can. Depending on your height and the health of your lower back, you will need to squat, sit, or bend at the waist, or use a chair. Point his body so that his penis aims down toward the water. Say a little prayer and start squeezing, adjusting your aim according to the "feedback" (that is, urine spraying all over the walls and floor) that you receive. Wipe up and resolve to improve with every squeeze. (Don't tell my houseguests, but I practiced with the guest room bathtub. Dr. Christman practiced with a sink, but he won't say which one.)

A few other notes on boys:

- If your dog has a little bit of muscular function, you may only need to get him started with a gentle squeeze before he takes over and does the rest. Just check to ensure the bladder is empty after he has finished.
- Sometimes the urine will spurt in pulses rather than flow, especially if the dog still has a little neurological function. This is normal and not a cause for worry.
- You may notice a short gap of time—a second or two—between your squeeze and the flow, as the urine makes the crazy straw turn.

risks — guess what? bladder rupture isn't one of them

From the Desk of Dr. Christman

A ruptured bladder is every paraplegic dog owner's paranoia. Don't worry. I highly doubt this will ever happen. In fact, I've never seen it in my practice. The urinary bladder is designed to stretch and distend as needed, because of those special cells, transitional cell epithelium, that the bladder is made of.

Why should you care? While it is technically possible for a dog's bladder to rupture from being too full, this is highly unlikely. For a rupture to happen, the bladder would have to be ignored for more than 24 hours and not be able to overflow for some reason to release the pressure.

I suppose it is possible that a rupture could result from pressing too hard, but that would require pressure more like a blow, not the firm but gentle steady compression used to express a bladder.

Overflow is still a problem, though.

Don't interpret this to mean that a constantly full bladder is okay. Delaying bladder expression too long will result in bladder overflow in the short term, and damage to the bladder and kidneys in the long term (see table at right). If you are expressing the bladder three to four times a day, you do not need to worry about these risks.

—Adam Christman, DVM, MBA

Dr. Christman's Guide: Risks of an Overflowing Bladder

Short-term Risks	Long-term Risks
Mess: Bladder overflow is inconvenient for you—it causes a mess. Dirty floors, smelly laundry. **Urine scald:** If your dog's skin is exposed to urine for long periods (for example, from lying on a blanket soaked in overflowed urine), her skin will be irritated by the caustic components. See page 100 for more information.	**Decreased bladder tone:** Like any stretchy material, the lining of the bladder can eventually lose its elasticity if it remains stretched for too long for too often. When a bladder loses tone, it is more likely to leak. Over several years, reduced tone can lead to actual incontinence. **Pre-renal azotemia:** A bladder filled to capacity can back up into the kidneys, eventually causing a harmful effect known as pre-renal azotemia, which means high nitrogen-containing compounds in the blood. This in turn means that the kidneys are not able to filter the blood properly. The symptoms are serious: vomiting, loss of appetite, lethargy, and restlessness. Seek veterinary attention if you know the bladder was not expressed for a long period and you see these signs. **Uremia and kidney failure:** Untreated pre-renal azotemia can lead to uremia, an excess of byproducts in the blood. These substances, like urea and creatinine, should be excreted in the urine. Uremia is an indication of kidney failure.

leaks are your fault, but you're still a good person

I know it's not fashionable these days to say that anything is someone's fault. Everyone wants their participation trophy. But here's the reality: If your paraplegic dog leaks, it's your fault.

The vast majority of the time, a leak is an overflow (the rest of the time, it probably indicates a urinary tract infection). An overflow happens when you don't regulate the water *intake* with the urine *output*. The beauty of realizing this: It means you can control it. You can control when the fluids go in, and you can control when the fluids go out. Remember, these dogs are not incontinent. The urine won't come out on its own unless the volume of urine in the bladder creates enough pressure to force it out.

You control when your dog drinks water. I am not saying you should ever withhold water. *You should not withhold water.* But you can encourage your dog to drink in small, frequent amounts, rather than in large, infrequent amounts. Put a little water on your dog's food. Tempt her with a few tablespoons of broth. When you make a tuna sandwich, give her that little bit of juice from the can. In the summertime, freeze yogurt or watermelon pieces for her to lick. There are lots of ways to get fluid into her a little at a time, which will help her urinary tract to stay on an even keel.

You control when you express the bladder. You know the drill by now: Express the bladder three to four times a day. As soon as you get up, as soon as you get home from work, and right before bed. More often if you can. You will have very few leaks if you keep to a regular, predictable schedule. If you notice that your dog has had a big drink of water, set your timer for an hour and do an extra squeeze when the alarm goes off.

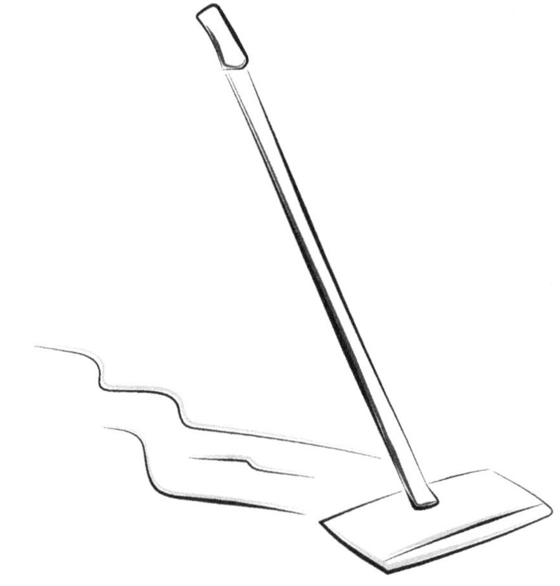

Be realistic, and be forgiving. I'm not saying leaks will never happen, and I'm not saying you should beat yourself up over a leak when it does. It doesn't make you a jerk. It will happen once in a while. Clean up, and move forward. You're still a good person. That's what mops are for.

urinary tract infections in paraplegic dogs

From the Desk of Dr. Christman

Urinary tract infections (UTIs) can be common in paraplegic dogs. Let's understand the two basic types of UTIs: lower and upper. Most UTIs start out as the lower type. These are infections of the bladder and urethra. An upper UTI is more dangerous, as these infections affect the kidneys. If you hear someone say "ascending UTI," they are talking about a lower UTI that spread upward to the kidneys. These upper UTIs can really do some damage if left untreated.

My three simple tips (at right) can minimize the risk of both types.

—Adam Christman, DVM, MBA

> **Girls and UTIs**
>
> UTIs can be more common in female IVDD dogs for two reasons:
>
> 1. The proximity of their urethra to the rectum increases the chance of exposure to fecal matter, which often contains e. coli, a common UTI bacteria.
> 2. The way they scurry on the floor may inoculate their urethra with bacteria.

Dr. Christman's First Tip: Express Fully

The most important—and the easiest—thing you can do to reduce the risk of UTI is to empty your dog's bladder completely every time you express it. Expressing the bladder fully cuts your risk of UTI significantly because it minimizes the opportunity for urine to become stagnant. Urine that lingers in the bladder can create an ideal environment for bacteria to grow. Since paraplegic dogs are less mobile than other dogs, their urine is especially likely to stagnate. When you squeeze that bladder, get it down to the very last drop.

Dr. Christman's Second Tip: Use Your Eyes and Nose

Normal urine is clear, straw-colored, and slightly acidic. It has the odor of urea. Its normal constituents include water, urea, sodium chloride, potassium chloride, phosphates, uric acid, organic salts, and the pigment urobilin.

Abnormal constituents indicative of disease include ketone bodies, protein, bacteria, blood, glucose, pus, and certain crystals. Some of these you may be able to see or smell; others you will not. Abnormal urine may be cloudy, and its pH may be more alkaline.

Since you are regularly expressing the bladder, you'll have a front-row seat to the color, clarity, and smell of your dog's urine. If you ever notice an unusual smell while you are expressing the bladder, or if the color is darker or lighter than the straw color for more than one day, ask your veterinarian for a urinalysis right away.

Dr. Christman's Third Tip: Urinalysis Twice a Year

Most dogs with a UTI will show obvious symptoms: accidents in the house, straining to urinate, or urinating frequent, small volumes. A paraplegic dog never has the opportunity to show these signs because you are expressing her bladder for her.

To keep a proactive eye on your dog's urinary tract health, I advise scheduling a urinalysis twice a year to make sure no overt infection is present. If you can detect a lower UTI early, before it ascends to the kidneys and becomes an upper UTI, it is much less likely to cause long-term trouble.

the golden fluid: earning your pee-h-d

From the Desk of Dr. Christman

Urine is what we veterinarians call "the golden fluid." It tells us a tremendous amount about an animal's overall health. What I am about to tell you is probably way more than you actually need to know about the chemistry of your dachshund's urine, but I think it's pretty interesting, and I thought you might too.

Two major urine tests (outlined below) give us a massive amount of information about the health of the dog's kidneys, bladder, and urethra: urinalysis and urine culture.

—Adam Christman, DVM, MBA

Dr. Christman's Guide to IVDD Urine Testing

Urinalysis

Most general practice vets can do a urinalysis in house, using three methods:

1. Visual check of color, cloudiness, and concentration:
    - **Color:** Normal urine will be straw-colored yellow. Darker urine is probably more concentrated, and lighter urine is diluted. If there is blood in the urine, it can be a red-brown color.
    - **Cloudiness:** May mean that the dog has an infection, and white blood cells are causing the urine to cloud.
    - **Concentration:** The specific gravity gives the exact concentration of the urine and indicates how well the kidneys are working.
2. Chemical analysis: Vets use a dipstick that has been divided into sections, each section with its own little pad. The pads test for different substances in the urine and change color when those substances are present. The most thorough dipsticks include eight or more tests. Examples include pH, protein, glucose, and blood, all indicating different types of disease, like diabetes, stones, or kidney disease.

3. Microscope exam of sediment: The veterinarian will put a bit of the sample through a centrifuge and examine the sediment that settles out under a microscope. The veterinarian looks for white blood cells, bacteria, crystals, and casts. These give the vet a lot of information about possible infections, inflammation, stones, and kidney health.

In a dog with IVDD, examining the golden fluid is especially useful, so I recommend two urinalyses per year just to keep on top of potential issues before they become problems.

Urine Culture

If your veterinarian sees evidence of infection during the urinalysis, they will likely recommend that you send a sterile urine sample to a lab for a urine culture. The culture identifies two things: exactly what bacteria is infecting the urinary tract, and exactly what antibiotic will resolve those infections. A culture, although a bit more expensive than the urinalysis, gives you a much better chance of actually resolving an infection on the first try.

The vet will draw a sample directly from the bladder with a needle to ensure it is not contaminated. The lab will use a special type of slide to encourage the bacteria to grow so they can identify it. This usually takes two to three days. Finally, the lab does sensitivity tests to identify which antibiotics will treat that specific bacteria.

Without the culture, the veterinarian can only guess at what antibiotic will work. Many vets will try a broad-spectrum antibiotic first, and then send a sample for culturing if the symptoms don't seem to be getting better.

poops you can be proud of

You may be thinking, "This has been a lot of pee talk. What about the poop?"

Good news! The poop is really different from the pee. (Boy, I never imagined I would write that sentence.) The biggest difference (besides the obvious) is that poop will come out on its own, without your help. There is no risk of it staying inside, causing infection or other damage, as there is with urine (unless you have something else going on besides IVDD).

Let me say that again: The digestive tract will push that poop on out. It may not come out when you want it to, or where you want it to, but it will come out. So, you have a couple of choices in your "poop attitude": the *Free to Be You and Me* hippie attitude or the *OCD Controlling* attitude.

Free to Be You and Me

If you are a live-and-let-live, freewheeling type, all you need to do is stock up on recycled paper towels and your favorite organic vinegar floor spray. When your dog poops, pick it up, hum a little Grateful Dead, and spritz around some patchouli essential oil room freshener. Then light a candle.

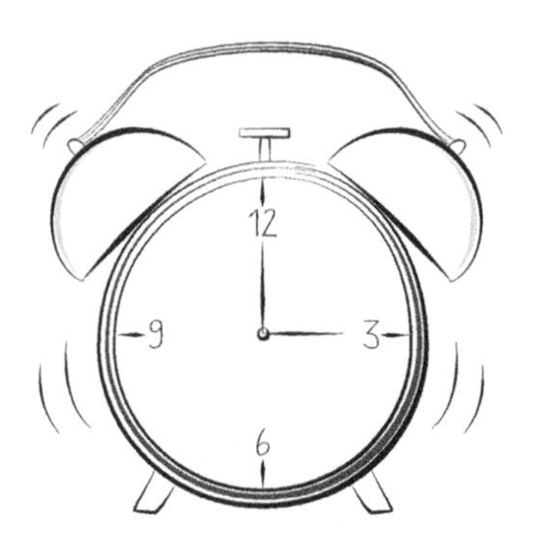

OCD Controlling

If you are more of an OCD type who requires control over the times and places you handle poop in your daily life, we are going to need a brief canine anatomy lesson.

The bowel and rectum run right below the spine, and right above the bladder. If all of this were on a map, Bowel Road would run parallel to Spine Highway, right above the very picturesque Bladder Pond.

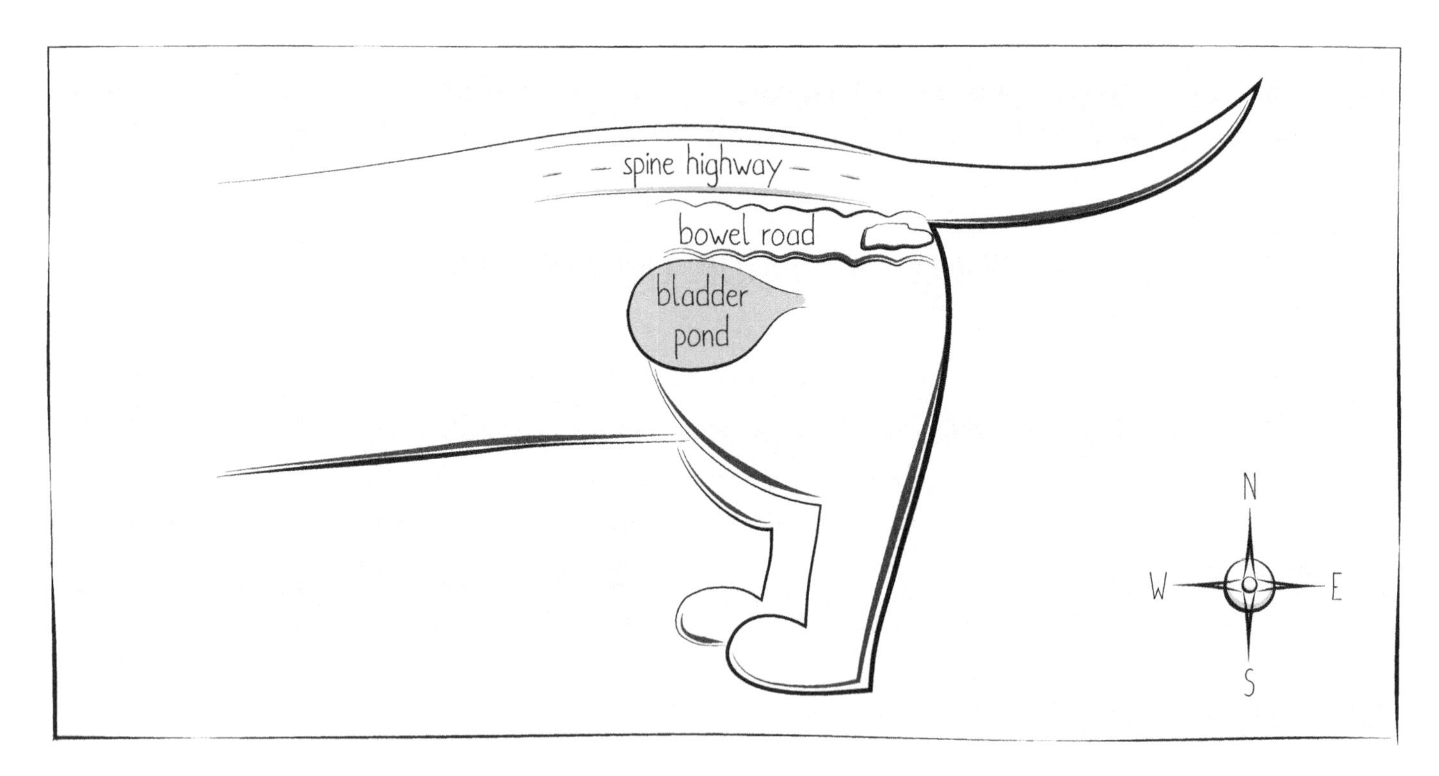

Approach the Poop!

You can approach the poop from below, you can approach it from above, or you can approach it from behind.

- **From below:** When in position to express the bladder, move your fingers up toward the spine and feel for the bowel. You will feel a solid, but not hard, substance. That's not a tumor—that's the poop! Squeeze the poop toward the rectum.[16]
- **From above:** Use your index finger and thumb to feel around the spine, a couple of inches forward from the base of the tail. If the poop is ready, you will feel something more solid than the rest of the abdomen, but not as hard as the bones of the spine. Squeeze it out. (This technique is especially easy if IVDD caused profound damage to the spinal cord, because there will be no muscle tone to get in the way of feeling the poop in the bowel.)
- **From behind:** Twirl a lubed Q-tip just inside the anus. In a few seconds, voila! The action will begin. This technique works best for dogs that still have some muscle tone in their anus (aka anal tone). Simple test: If she puckers her anus when you put the Q-tip in, your dog has anal tone.

Bonus: Getting the poop out sometimes makes expressing the bladder easier, because poop in the rectum can slow down the urine flow by pressing on the urethra. (True for some dogs, not true for others.)

Avoid the Runs. At All Costs, Avoid the Runs!

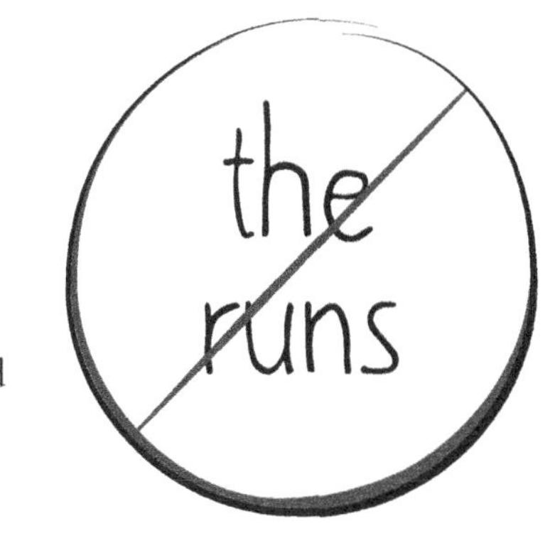

If you keep a keen eye on your paraplegic dog's diet, using the same food and treats every day, your dog is less likely to experience intestinal distress. Intestinal distress—a nice way to say "the runs"—is no fun with a paraplegic dog. No fun at all. (Imagine a normal dog with diarrhea. Now imagine a paraplegic dog with it: laundry on the "Shit Storm" washer setting, undignified dog-bathing followed by highly unpleasant tub-washing, and a scalding hot shower for you—in other words, every last ounce of hot water in the house.)

Consistency of diet is the key to your sanity. If you find that even with consistent diet, your dog's poops are generally a bit soft, experiment with higher-fiber food. Or add some fiber to your dog's diet. All you need for easy-peasy poops is a little psyllium husk, or a teaspoon or two of canned pure pumpkin. Keep the diet very, very simple. Your goal: nice, neat, tidy poops you can be proud of.

---

[16] The first time I felt the rectum this way, I rushed Tabby to the veterinarian because I thought she had a tumor. The veterinarian gently informed me, "Oh, that's just BM." That's how I discovered this technique. Thank you, Dr. Matthew Miller!

From the Desk of Dr. Christman

The digestive tract is motivated by involuntary muscular contractions called peristalsis. These contractions still happen in paraplegic dogs. That's why the paraplegic dog can still digest her food normally, and why paraplegic dogs can poop on their own, even though most cannot control the timing.

Occasionally I find my dachshund dropping what I call "nuggets." He doesn't know he's doing it. He's just shimmying around the house or yard in his usual way, conducting his doggie investigations and generally having a good time.

To control Cosmo's nugget production, I press near his perirectal region and gently milk out the fecal balls over the toilet. Works like a charm. With a bit of practice, you too will have your paraplegic dog's urinary and fecal outputs down to a science.

If you want what comes out of your dog to be easily manageable, however, you need to manage what goes in. You always want your paraplegic dog to have nicely formed stool, not diarrhea and not constipation.

Consistent diet and adequate water are very important.

Maintaining a consistent diet is paramount for a paraplegic dog. You want them to have nicely formed stool, and you want them to stay lean so they do not have to drag around extra weight. Of course, you also want them to receive the essential nutrients they need.

I keep Cosmo on a premium weight-managed commercial dog food. I use a weight-management formulation because I know he's not going to burn as many calories as he did before his rupture, unless I take him swimming or put him in his cart. I use a premium food that I researched, so I know it has the nutrients Cosmo needs. Because I want Cosmo's "nuggets" to be nice and formed, I make sure that his food has an adequate amount of fiber (about 4 percent).

It is always important to make sure your dog has clean, cool water at all times. In addition to bladder and kidney issues, lack of water can cause constipation.

—Adam Christman, DVM, MBA

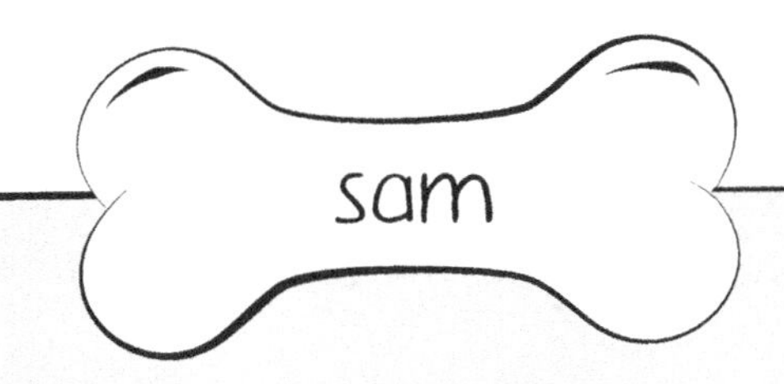

Because of Sam...

Every now and then, something happens that, even though you don't really want to be part of it, you are drawn to it. That was the case with Sam, a piebald dachshund. Sam had a family, but when he was four years old, he became paralyzed. His family took him to the vet, where he was diagnosed with IVDD and sent home with meds and instructions for crate rest and bladder expression. After about a week, the family decided it was too much to care for Sam and surrendered him to rescue. I became his foster mom. I gave him his meds, expressed his bladder, and took him to his vet appointments and therapies. It was obvious to everyone but me that I was falling in love, and my family decided to adopt Sam.

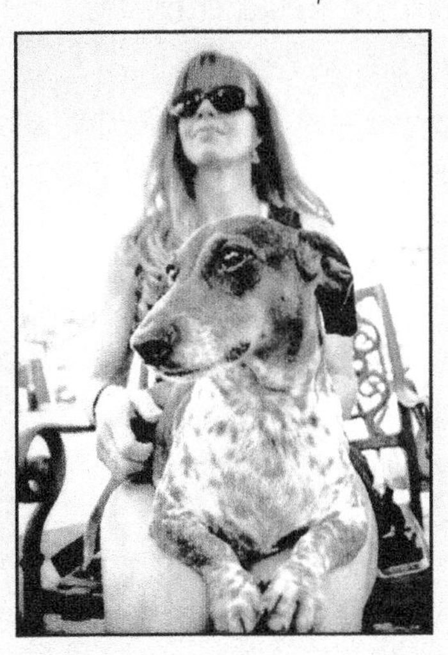

Sam became a master scooter. He can get around the house and yard as quickly as any other dog. He loves to go for walks in his cart, and he drinks in the attention he gets from our neighbors. With physical therapy, Sam regained bowel and bladder control, plus the ability to take four to five steps at a time with "spinal walking," now his primary source of mobility. That's good enough for us!

Because of Sam, I got heavily involved in rescue. Because of Sam, I've helped find numerous dogs new homes, I've helped find carts for families who can't afford them for their paralyzed pets, and I've transported dogs to rescues, adoptive homes, and foster homes. Because of Sam, I've done countless home visits to help find foster dogs their forever homes and counseled many people on what to do when their dogs become paralyzed. Because of Sam, I started a fundraiser to help the rescues that so desperately need money to keep saving lives.

Words cannot describe the joy Sam has brought me, and a whole new appreciation for the imperfect, the unwanted—because those are the most rewarding, most appreciative, most loving. I love to share this story to inspire others to adopt (or keep) the imperfect ones. Because of Sam, my family is complete.

—Kelly Maxwell (Port Orange, Florida)

mighty max

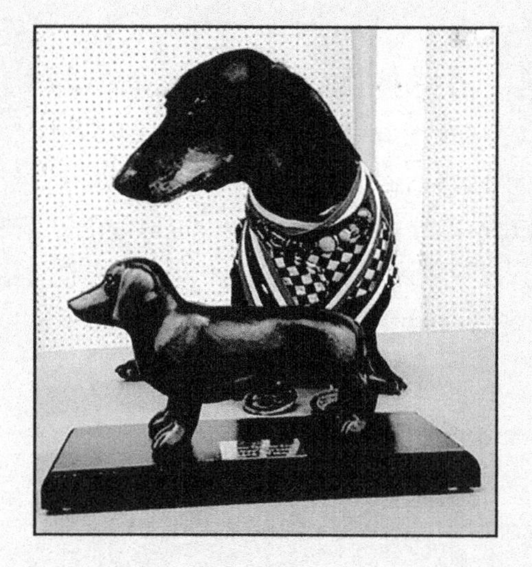

Little Mighty Max is always wanting to please, never getting into any trouble, and very laid back...until he gets to a race.

Not long after I adopted Max, I learned about the dachshund races, and a few weeks later we were on our way to Atlanta to compete in the races at Howl-O-Weenie, DREAM Dachshund Rescue's annual dachshund festival. I decided to enter Max in the wheelie race and see if it was something he would enjoy. His first race was only two weeks after he got his new wheels. At first, he was in the lead, but he made a U-turn to go back for a hot dog that someone had dropped on the field during the dunking contest. Still, I could tell by his attitude that racing was something he loved to do. His next race was at the Georgia Dachshund Races the following summer. He won, and since then he has been hooked, winning his next four in a row! When Max sees he is at a race, he will puff up his chest and get a strut in his walk. He loves wearing his medals—sometimes he tells me that he wants me to put his medals around his neck so he can wear them while he relaxes on the couch and watches TV.

Mighty Max is also a bit of a fashionista. He loves picking out an outfit, and he loves wearing hats! Mighty Max is such a joy. Adopting him has been the best decision of my life.

—Amanda Beeler (Knoxville, Tennessee)

the down-dog-friendly home and yard

Inside

- Smooth floors—tile, linoleum, laminate, or hardwood
- Baby gates separating them from carpet, which can be abrasive on the skin. (Luckily, they don't need to be very tall gates.)
- Ramps for sliding down off the bed/couch
- Lots of beds and blankies that are easy to wash
- Chair by the toilet for you
- Antibacterial soap

Outside

- Grassy yard for chasing squirrels. They still like to play and go outside with their buddies, even to chase squirrels (though not as frequently successful)
- Limited access to rough surfaces like scratchy pavestones or concrete
- Ramp from porch or deck (alternative: ready human for carrying). They are unlikely to be able to pull themselves up a ramp, but they sure love sliding down them!

Other Tips

- Pet sitter 1: A pet sitter who you trained to express your dog's bladder—and who was then able to put "special needs dogs" on their website
- Pet sitter 2: Vet tech from your veterinarian's office

skin concerns

FIRST AID

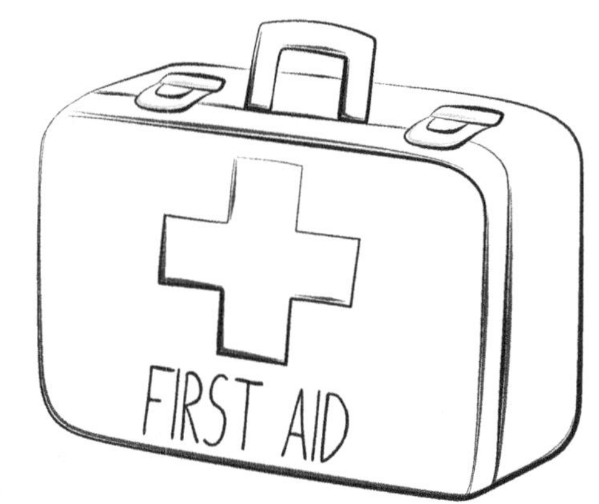

When people meet my down dogs at the park, one of the first things they ask is whether their skin gets hurt from dragging around. (These questions come after the obligatory, "Oh, that's so sad!" remarks, which my girls quickly change their minds about by scooting merrily past in the background chasing after a ball or another dog. Double-takes abound.)

It's a valid question, of course. For my small dogs (ranging from eight to thirteen pounds), it just hasn't been an issue. For a larger paraplegic dog, the skin is much more of a serious concern, but most dachshunds do not have enough weight pressing on the skin to cause pressure problems.

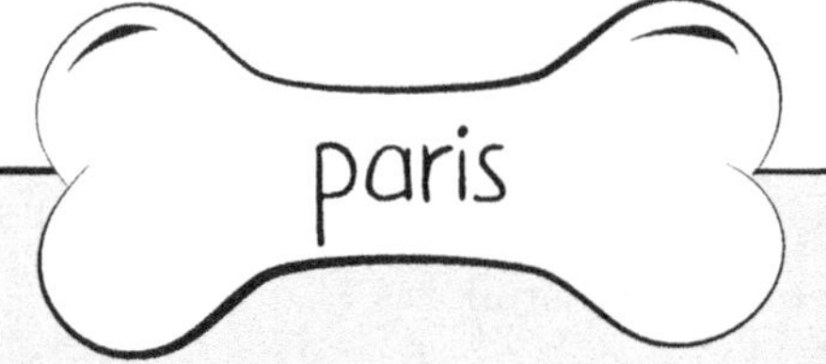

paris

IF MOM DOESN'T
COME WHEN I CALL,
I HURL MYSELF
DOWN THESE STAIRS.
even though I'm paraplegic.

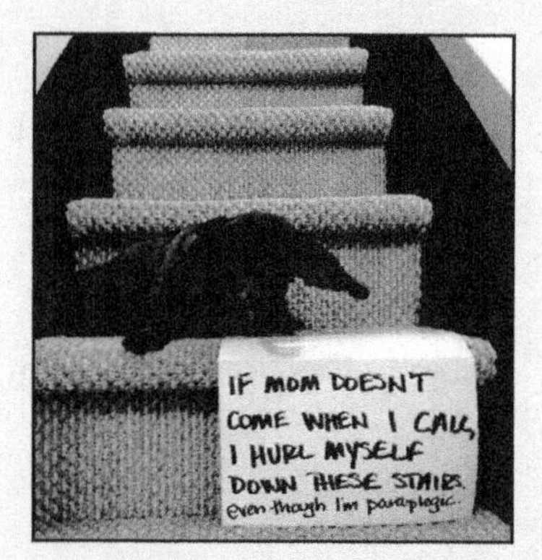

Paris was five years old when she had a profound disc rupture and came to rescue with no use of her back legs. Her owner had waited too long to get her surgery. The rescue tried crate rest with medications, but her spinal cord damage was permanent. She never regained any function.

Being paralyzed has never stopped Paris from having adventures. Whenever she sees a suitcase get packed, she positions herself by the front door so she can hurl herself down the front steps and try to go on the trip too. She is the oldest dog in her pack and bullies everyone around her—her best trick is to position herself at the top of the ramp to the bed so that when the other dogs try to come up, she can act like the troll under the bridge from the fairy tale. She also chases chickens. Paris is now 10 years old.

—Kristin Leydig Bryant

Small injuries are inevitable, so you should be aware of a few ways your down dachshund's skin could get hurt. *Be sure to keep a doggie first aid kit on hand, and you should be able to deal with any little boo-boos.*

Abrasions

The most common skin problem comes from rubbing over rough surfaces. Obviously, a dog with tender skin exposed to the ground should not be dragging it across concrete or asphalt. If you want to take your dog for a walk on a paved street or sidewalk, use a wheelchair cart or a sling. I usually just take mine to an enclosed grassy area and let them enjoy themselves. They follow me around until something (squirrel!) distracts them, and then they take off for a bit of adventure. They even join in the other dogs' games of chase (although not very successfully).

Carpet Burns

You can avoid rug burn irritation by not giving your dog access to carpeted areas. Just crossing a throw rug is fine. But if your dog is pulling herself across carpet for longer periods, check her belly to make sure she isn't inflamed.

Ear Itchies

From the Desk of Dr. Christman

It may surprise you to realize that the ears are a bit of a problem for paraplegic dogs. Not because IVDD affects the ears, but because these dogs cannot use their rear legs to scratch like other dogs do. The ability to scratch serves two purposes: It is how your dog relieves an itch, and it's how you notice that there might be a problem.

Most of my patients with ear infections came to my office because their owners noticed them scratching their ears. This will not be the case with a down dog. They may have the itch, but you won't see the scratch.

To make sure my paralyzed dachshund's ears are in good shape and comfortable, I check Cosmo's ears regularly. I help him with his itchies every day with a good scratch session, and I clean his ears every week to prevent ear infections, watching carefully for signs of irritation, discharge, or excessive waxy buildup.

—Adam Christman, DVM, MBA

Urine Scald

Prolonged contact with urine can irritate a dog's skin, just like diaper rash on a human baby. The caustic components of urine can be especially damaging to the tender skin of the genitals and belly, which don't have as much protective hair covering. You can soothe these burns with anti-inflammatory/antibiotic creams or coconut oil. But prevention is even easier—express the bladder at regular intervals, and give a good wash down in case of a leak. Keep some baby wipes handy, and if you see any irritation of your dog's skin, take care of it before an infection sets in.

From the Desk of Dr. Christman

If a dog's skin is in contact with urine for more than 48–72 hours—usually from wet bedding or a diaper—she will likely develop urine scald. When scalding happens, the skin is "burned" by the urinary pH altering the skin's pH. Urine scald can cause redness, infection, and hair loss to the skin exposed to the urine. You may also see a moist discharge.

Incontinent dogs can leak small quantities of urine while resting or sleeping. Most IVDD dogs, however, are not truly incontinent. Leaks in an IVDD-paralyzed dog most often result from the owner not fully expressing the bladder, or waiting too long between expressions, causing an overflow.

IVDD dogs are more prone to UTIs, so their urine is also more likely to be concentrated and/or alkaline. Urine like this is more likely to cause urine scald.

If your dog seems to have a minor case of scald, you can treat it with over-the-counter topical antibiotic and corticosteroid creams. Use an Elizabethan collar or other device to preventing her from licking the area.

If these methods do not clear up her skin within a week, seek veterinary care. She probably needs an oral antibiotic and/or a corticosteroid injection. In severe cases, urine scald can lead to a septicemia (blood-borne bacterial infection) that can make your dog very sick.

—Adam Christman, DVM, MBA

Diapers

Many paraplegic dog owners use diapers, but I'm not a big fan of them, personally. Diapers can exacerbate urine scalding, as they hold the fluid in contact with the skin. I also think it's important for you to be able to see your dog's rear end, so you can make sure it's clean and without any signs of irritation or infection. If you're squeezing the bladder correctly and often enough, your dog should not need a diaper.

Lichenification (Elephant Tail)

Since many paralyzed dogs scoot with their tails tucked under their butts, you may see the hair getting worn away and not growing back. This is usually just cosmetic, but it's a good idea to ask your veterinarian to rule out other causes (unrelated to IVDD).

From the Desk of Dr. Christman

On many dachshunds, but especially on "down" dachshunds, you may see a thickening of the skin of the tail until it becomes elephant-like. This leathery skin usually results from constant rubbing, but it can also happen on skin that doesn't get that friction (much like male pattern baldness in human men). Lichenification also commonly occurs on dachshunds' ears, but this of course is not related to their IVDD. A paraplegic dog's tail spends a lot of time rubbing across the floor as the dog shimmies around. The hair just disappears. When the hair loss reaches a certain point, it generally gets no worse.

Lichenification is sort of a non-problem; simply a cosmetic issue. If you see what you believe is lichenification, ask your veterinarian to check it out to eliminate the possibility of other skin problems like folliculitis or eczema. You should not see flaking or sores. There are no other health problems associated with lichenification in dachshunds.

—Adam Christman, DVM, MBA

Pressure Sores

If your paralyzed dog is allowed to scoot around the house during the day, pressure sores (also known as bed sores) are unlikely, because her body weight will not press on one part of her body for a prolonged period. Allow freedom of movement, encourage your dog to be active, and make sure she is not overweight.

From the Desk of Dr. Christman

Pressure sores, also known as hygromas, can happen in any down dog, but are more common in the larger to giant breed dogs. My Cosmo has had very mild pressure sores on the outside of his hocks and on the top of his tail. I have very rarely had to use any topicals on him. A thick layer of clean, dry bedding and lots of blankets will help prevent pressure sores. You can also encourage your dog to sleep (and nap!) on different sides every day.

—Adam Christman, DVM, MBA

What All of This Means

If you keep your doxie on the thin side to minimize weight on her tummy, don't let her drag across anything rough, and keep her clean, you shouldn't need to worry about her skin too much..

COSMO

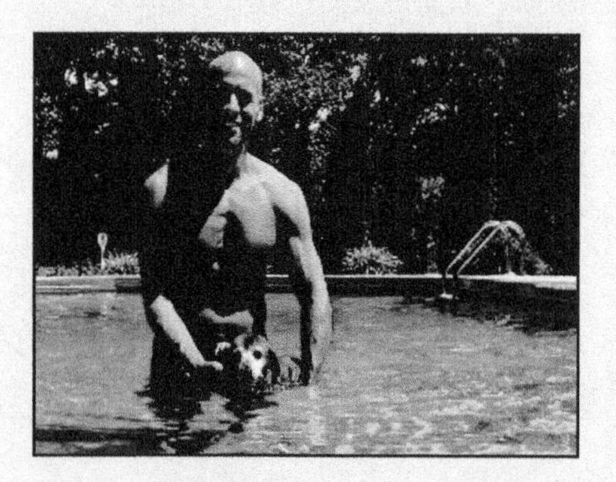

Every spring, when we open our backyard pool, I tell Cosmo, "Cosmo, the pool is opening today!" and he goes crazy! He waits until I have the water balanced, and then he goes shimmying off to where I store his life jacket. Once he hears the click of the jacket buckle, he is ready to swim! He loves the pool. All of my friends and family adore swimming with him. He has his own umbrella and water dish on the deck, and he loves relaxing with anyone who will give him room on a swim float.

Cosmo went down at the age of two. He is now 13 years old.

—Adam Christman, DVM, MBA

part five: rollin', rollin', rollin' — wheelchair carts

Cue the "Rawhide" music! It's time to think about a wheelchair cart! Do you need one? When? What kind? And how do you get started?

Do you really need a cart?

Many down dachshunds are perfectly happy pulling themselves around the house, doing their own particular version of the IVDD Shimmy. If your home has smooth floors, and you don't plan to take your dog out on the open road, you may not need a cart at all.

A cart isn't necessary for hanging around the house, snuggling, or even exploring the grassy yard. A cart can be a real spirit-lifter for some dogs but unimportant to others, depending on the personality, age, and general life priorities of your dachshund.

Why would a dog want a cart?

The two main reasons for wanting a cart are Mobility and Protection.

1. Mobility: If your dachshund lives for walkies, a cart is the bee's knees. She will love zipping around the neighborhood, park, or hiking trail in her cart. Some dogs can actually run faster with the cart than they could before IVDD.
2. Protection: A cart allows your dog to move around without dragging her skin on the floor (inside) or the ground (outside). If you want to walk her on a sidewalk or street, you don't want that tender belly to drag over a paved surface. If your home has carpeted or otherwise abrasive floors, a cart can protect her skin.

> I feel the need... the need for speed!

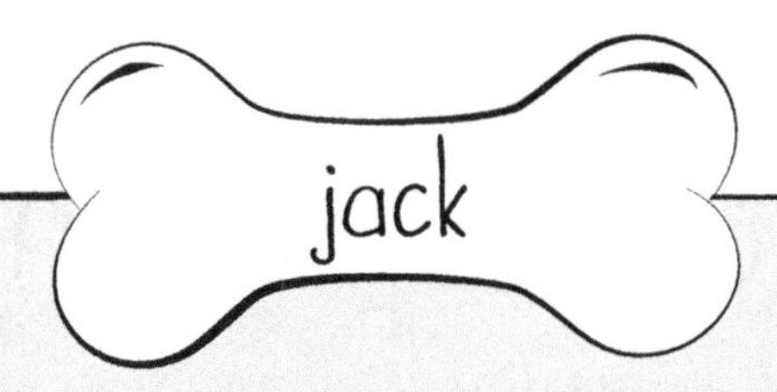

jack

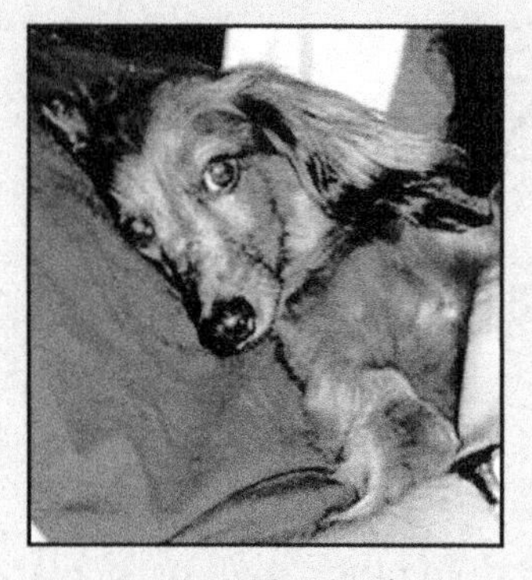

Jack's hunting instincts never dulled after his paralysis, even into old age. He would hide in the evenings under a bush in the backyard, waiting for his prey to emerge. One night, his ambush went beyond even his wildest dreams. I heard an otherworldly screeching and went flying out the back door to find Jack in mortal combat with an abnormally large squirrel, the creature's head entirely in Jack's mouth. Jack weighed only 11 pounds, and when I scooped him up, the squirrel was dangling from Jack's mouth. He didn't release it. I was surprised to see the squirrel was almost as long as he was—and then I was horrified to see the long, skinny, bare tail and realize the "squirrel" was really a large rat! Jack had killed it when it ventured from the woodpile, and he wasn't going to let it go now. I yelled at my husband, "Bring some cheese to make a trade!" Craig returned with a stick of butter. Just as my mind registered, "Butter?" Jack let go of the rat and grabbed the butter. For days afterwards, I swear he had a swagger in his IVDD shimmy.

Jack went down at nine years old. I came home from work one afternoon, and he came running to greet me by putting his front paws on my knees, as he had done hundreds of times before. When he landed back on the floor, he was screaming and already paralyzed. Surgery was unsuccessful in restoring the ability to walk. Jack had never been a determined sort of dog. He gave up on things easily. If he couldn't get to a toy, he would whine for it, rather than dig for it. If another dog stole his bed, he'd look at me to "fix it" rather than crowding in. He just wasn't a fighter. Unlike every other IVDD dog I've known, being paraplegic depressed him.

But when Jack got in his cart, he lit up. His daily walkies kept him alive. Every year, we would take him to the beach, strap that cart on, let him off leash, and he would fly, ears streaming behind him, far ahead of the other dogs. He loved to run, and the cart gave that back to him. He lived another six years before he died from causes unrelated to his IVDD.

—Kristin Leydig Bryant

when is it time to get a cart?

After your Base Treatment, the timing of getting a cart is a hugely subjective judgment call. Most carts are not therapeutic[17]—they do not assist in recovery. A cart is, however, super-fun for the dog. She can go in it—and she can go fast. Wheeee!

That Wheeee! can have one of two effects, depending on the attitude of your dog to start with:

> Don't even consider a cart until after you have completed your base treatment (surgery or crate rest). It's not time yet. You have plenty of other things to occupy your mind.

1. **Bad Wheeee!** Decreases motivation to learn to walk without the cart. The cart is easy, the cart is fast, the cart is fun—why should she bother with awkward regular walking with these slow legs? However, if you keep your cart sessions short, the increased mobility can actually be more motivating in the long term.
2. **Good Wheeee!** For dachshunds who become depressed by their reduced mobility, the freedom of movement of the cart can be a real picker-upper.

You will need to decide the best timing for getting a cart, if you do decide to get one.

My personal belief is that most dogs should not get a cart until they reach a plateau in recovery: They stall out. When your dog has stopped making regular progress after surgery or crate rest, it's time for a little boost. That's the time to introduce a cart. Or, if you think that some outside adventures would be beneficial for her state of mind, it's time to get the cart.

A lot depends on the personality of your dog.

[17] Exception: a walking cart, as discussed on page 110.

choosing a cart

There are three basic types of carts: customized metal, adjustable metal, and PVC (see table to the right). The customized metal ones are the most sophisticated, while the PVC ones are the simplest. Each has advantages and disadvantages over the others. Your choice will depend on how and where your dog wants to use the cart. See page 133 for the websites of some example manufacturers, as well as tips on finding a used cart or making your own cart. Please note that these are examples, not recommendations. My aim is to give you guidance on how to find the cart that suits your dog, your home, and your lifestyle.

Talk the Talk Before You Wheel the Walk

Your best bet is to talk to several people about their experiences before you buy. We have listed several supportive online communities on page 132. Talk to people who seem to have similar situations to yours. These folks love to talk to people about their dogs, and they love to help people like you.

In your forum post, start out by describing your dachshund's situation and personality, as well as how you'd like to be able to use the cart. After that, consider asking some of these questions:

- What is the best thing about the cart you chose?
- What, if anything, would you change about your cart?
- How hard is it to get your dog into the cart?
- How long has your dog been using the cart?
- Does the cart require any maintenance?

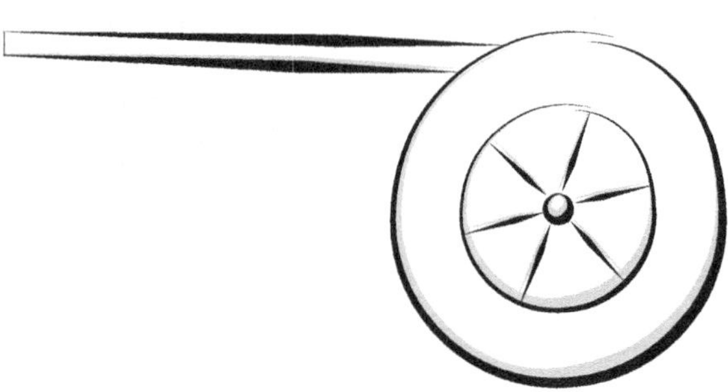

Then ask any specific questions about the features listed in the following table related to your situation and the cart manufacturers you are most interested in.

	Customized Metal Cart	Adjustable Metal Cart	PVC Cart
Stability	Very stable on almost all surfaces.	Very stable on many surfaces.	Stable only on even surfaces.
Wheelbase width	Most are quite wide.	Varies. Some styles are just as wide as the customized metal ones; others are narrower.	Tend to be narrow.
Weight	Tend to be heavier, but a young active dog will not notice. An older dog might have trouble.	Middleweight, probably suitable for all but a very old dog.	Lightweight.
Outdoor use	Good for hiking trails and other uneven terrain. Even works on gravel. Good for very active dogs who want to make quick turns at a run.	Good for somewhat uneven outdoor terrain or easy hiking trails. May tip over on a quick turn or on a hill or curb.	Good for smooth sidewalks or road. A dog can get a great run going on an even road or beach, but it can tip over easily on an uneven surface. A quick turn will probably result in a spill.
Indoor use	The wide wheelbase makes these carts less suitable for inside, as the dog is very prone to getting stuck between the legs of furniture.	The narrow styles are good for inside.	Narrow wheelbase makes these the best for inside carts.
Seat: Saddle, rings, or bar?	Most have either a saddle (popular for Walking Carts) or stationary rings (popular for Suspension Carts).	These carts tend to provide a choice between the rings and the saddle.	Most use a bar to hold up the hindquarters.
Adjustability	Most have some adjustability, but are built for a specific dog's detailed measurements.	Built in standard sizes (XS, S, M, L, XL) that you adjust for your dog.	Custom-built to your dog's detailed measurements. Not adjustable without cutting and reassembly.
Cost	Generally highest cost, but great variability among these sellers.	Likely to be moderate cost.	Lowest cost.

Suspension Cart or Walking Cart?

A **suspension** cart is purely for mobility. These carts help your dog get around the house and yard, go on walkies, and basically have a great time showing off their newfound speed. They keep your dog's rear feet safely off the ground. If your dog's back feet knuckle over, her rear legs cross each other, or she is not showing signs of walking again, you want a suspension cart—at least, for now.

Much like an underwater treadmill, a **walking** cart gives your dog the opportunity to practice walking while supported by the cart. These carts are best for IVDD dogs who just have a bit of weakness in the rear legs, or dogs who have started making walking movements with their rear legs. They can be used for short rehabilitation sessions. If you get a walking cart, take great care that the rear feet are not injured on longer walks or rough surfaces.

Now, before you go all Type A on me again, thinking, "Walking cart all the way, baby!" remember this caveat: Paralyzed dogs should start out with a suspension cart. If needed, most carts can be converted from a suspension cart to a walking cart later.

Don't Stress the Back!

Make sure that the cart you choose will not put any pressure on the spine. You want your dachshund's back to remain level and horizontal. You do not want anything about the cart to put pressure on the back. Pay particular attention to the position of the yoke (if there is one). It should rest squarely on the shoulders, where the front legs can support its weight.

Ease of Use

Choose a cart that will be easy for you and easy for them. You want a cart that is simple to get your dog into and out of, and easy for your dog to tool around in. If the cart isn't easy for both of you, you are very unlikely to want to use it. None of us needs additional hassle, now do we?

Most of the customized metal carts fall into one of two types: Those with padded rings for the dog's rear legs, and those with a suspended saddle to support the dog from beneath. If your dog has some control of her back legs, but not quite enough to support her weight and walk, she may be happiest in a cart with a saddle. Saddles feel more natural and allow more normal range of motion. A saddle is preferable for a Walking Cart. If your dog is completely paralyzed, you may have an easier time getting her in and out of a Suspension Cart with the padded rings.

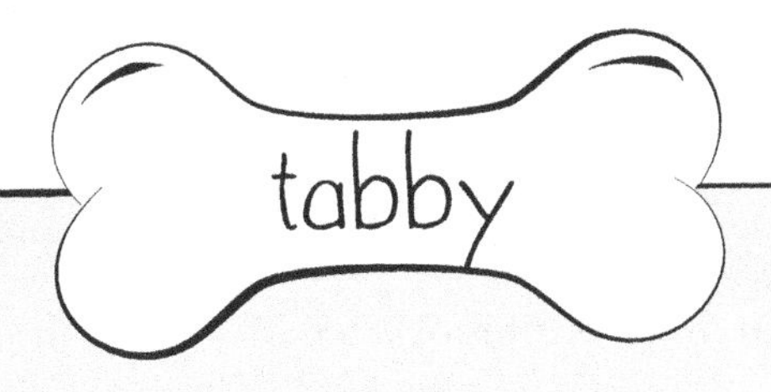

tabby

Photo by Regina Reif

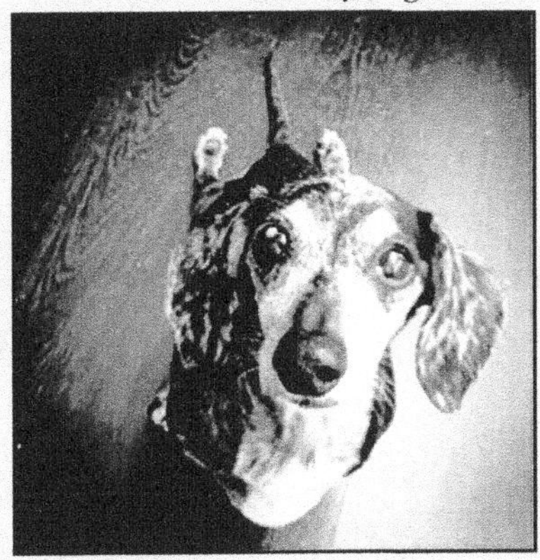

Craig and I would often marvel, "If Tabby could use all four legs, she would be a very bad dog." She was always into everything. She would steal any food she could reach—she once grabbed a lemon wedge out of my hand and swallowed it before she realized what it was. Another time, she filched a bag of rice out of the groceries before they were put away and dragged it to a corner to enjoy in secret. The next day, when I expressed her poop, I thought she had the worst case of tapeworms in history. Then I found her stash, the rice completely consumed except for a half-inch in the bottom of the shredded plastic. I've always imagined her thinking to herself, "I can do this! Just a few more grains!"

Tabby was a squeaky toy connoisseur. She would slide along the wooden floor like a slippery seal to chase her favorite, over and over and over, bringing the toy back again and again. She never got tired. If the toy had stuffing, she would gleefully eviscerate it until she was surrounded by clouds of white fuzz and a flat shell of plush.

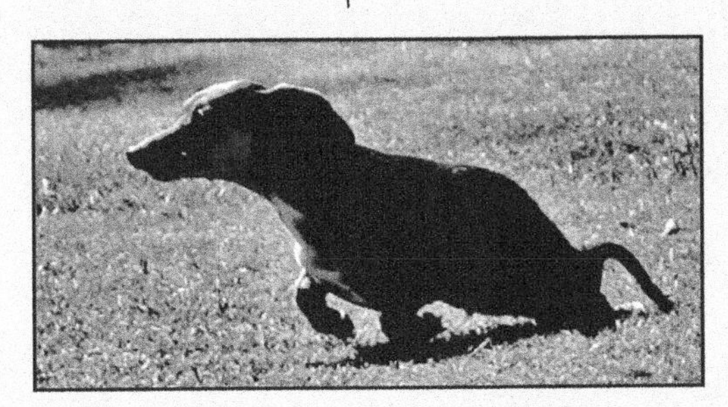

Tabby was the first paraplegic dachshund I ever knew. We learned together. She went down when she was six years old after escaping her owners' yard and going on a walkabout adventure (no surprise) that included jumping off a wall. Her family turned her in to rescue after they found the little fugitive paralyzed.

I adopted her after realizing she was my "dog of a lifetime." Tabby lived with us for 11 years after her disc rupture. She died at age 17 of causes unrelated to her IVDD.

—Kristin Leydig Bryant

used carts and DIY carts

Used Carts

When considering a used cart, keep in mind the importance of a good fit. If the cart is uncomfortable, your dog may not be willing or able to take any steps in it, defeating the whole purpose. Additionally, poor fit could cause other issues with your dog's back and legs. Make sure the cart fits and is comfortable for your dog, and that it's not putting any pressure on the back itself.

Occasionally, cart manufacturers will make used carts available to people with financial restrictions. You can also try http://useddogwheelchairs.com/, eBay, and Craigslist. People will often donate carts to dachshund rescues. (At one point, I had seven carts in my attic!) Contact your local rescue group and offer a donation in exchange for a cart.

DIY Carts

If you are a handy sort, search the Internet, especially for videos; type in "dog wheelchair design" to see several examples of make-at-home wheelchairs. Most designs use PVC or metal tubing as the structure. Many DIY-ers use the wheels from yard-sale baby strollers.

the cart has arrived! now what do i do?

The big day is here, and you're ready to see your dachshund zip around in her new wheels. Many dogs take off running as soon as you put them in the cart. Be prepared and have the leash on when you strap that baby in.

But some dogs don't quite catch on at first. If she doesn't take to it right away, double-check three things (as well as any instructions from your cart provider):

1. **Fit:** Is anything restricting her movements, especially in the front legs?
2. **Balance:** Is the cart pressing down on her back (or pulling it up)? The horizontal bar should be horizontal, and any straps should not be straining.
3. **Weight:** Is she physically able to pull the weight of the cart?

Fit, balance, and weight are critical. If they seem to be in order, she may need a bit of encouragement. And for most dachshunds, "encouragement" means "a treat."

Get a really, really valuable treat—something smelly. The stinkier, the better. Something she never gets otherwise. If it's offensive to your nose, it's probably good. Chicken baby food on the end of a spoon, for example. Or liverwurst. Or actual liver.

Find a comfortable, familiar area with no distractions. Strap her in the cart, and sit a few feet in front of her with the treat just tantalizingly out of her reach. Any time she takes a step, she gets one lick and huge, enthusiastic praise from you in your jolliest voice. Back up and do it again.

Do this for no more than five minutes, watching carefully to ensure you didn't miss any problems with fit, balance, or weight. (Short, happy training sessions ensure she won't build up a negative association with the cart. Keep things light and make it into a game.) If you are sure that the cart is a good match for her, continue these tempting treat sessions until she is running around joyfully.

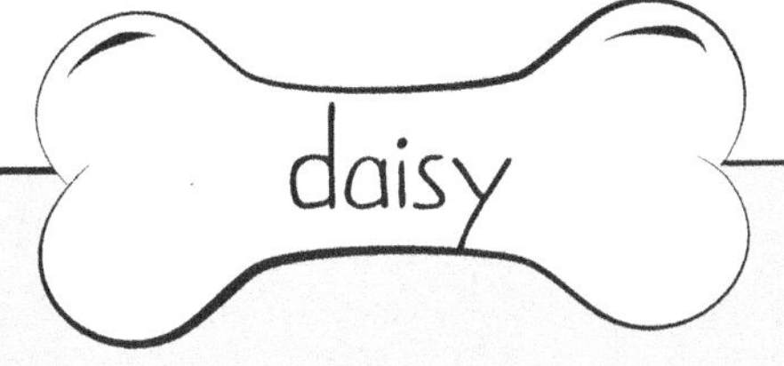

When I learned that the Florida Wiener Dog Derby would be in a nearby town instead of all the way at the other end of Florida, I signed both Daisy and Sam up for the wheelie dog division, appropriately titled Chariots of Fire. Daisy had been paralyzed since she was six years old.

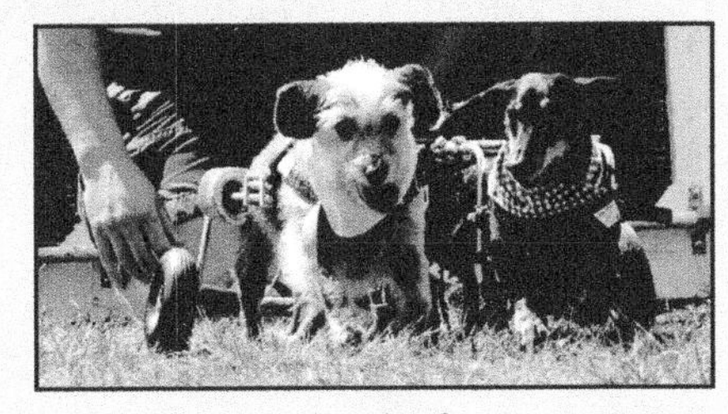

Race day came, and there were so many cart dogs that they had to run in multiple heats! My daughter Joanna was the "starting line" person, while I cheered them in at the finish line. Daisy was the first cart dog to cross the finish line in her heat, and then she won a medal for coming in second overall in the Chariots of Fire finals!

The following year, Daisy was to defend her title. She was once again the second overall finisher in the Chariots of Fire division. A true champion! As a result, the Florida Wiener Dog Derby invited Daisy to be a part of their team when they performed at the half-time show for the Orlando Predators!

— Kelly Maxwell (Port Orange, Florida)

brea & blossom

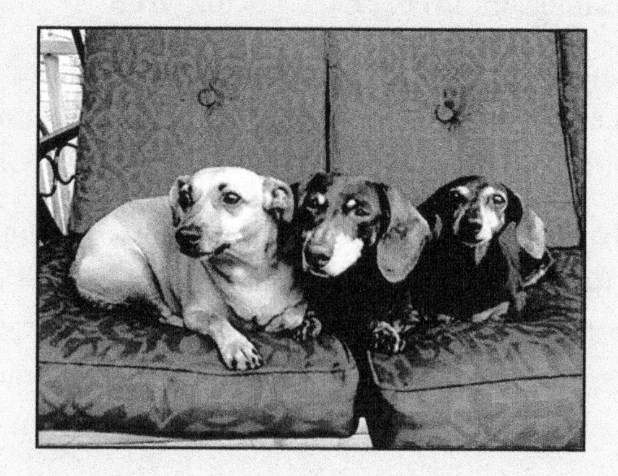

When we think of our crazy wheelie doxies, we think of their spunk and the fact that they don't "know" they are paralyzed. Brea went down when she was about eight, and Blossom was paralyzed at the age of five. We also have two "able-bodied" dogs, and sometimes they cannot keep up with Brea and Blossom. Since they cannot jump, we place them on the couch when we want to sit for any time. When we get up even for a second, Brea barks incessantly as if to say, "Don't forget about me! Let me off the couch! I know I'm not allowed to jump!" Blossom, on the other hand, just goes for it. She still loves to jump and "run," and she is often too fast for us to catch! She loves to fake a "damsel in distress" when she doesn't want to have to navigate across the slippery kitchen floor by herself. When she sees treats on the other end of the kitchen, though, she is magically able to scoot herself along rather quickly. (Funny how that works!)

Today, Brea is almost 15 and Blossom is 11. They both love to swim in our backyard pool. They just need lifejackets and are ready to go. Brea's latest funny habit is to be the "crazy old lady who says whatever she wants." She is almost 15 and will not slow down for anything. She knows the cabinet where we keep their cranberry dog treats. Whenever I go into the cabinet for any reason, she barks and barks and barks until I give her a treat.

—Susan and Eddie Womack (Douglasville, Georgia)

What If She Doesn't Like It?

If she really doesn't want to use the cart, don't force it. Try again in a couple of weeks, or in a different place. My current paraplegic dachshunds prefer to go au naturel and just thump thump thump to wherever they want to go. They wrestle, play, and chase balls that way. That is their choice. If they are happy, I'm happy.

Tips on Using the Cart

A cart is not meant for 24/7 use. Let your dachshund show you how long and how often she wants to use the cart. Most dogs should be in the cart for only a couple of hours at a time on a typical day.

Inside

- Put your dog in the cart only when you are home. Some dogs have trouble using the cart inside because they get stuck between furniture legs or on doorways as they tool around the house.
- Take the cart off before bedtime. The cart limits your dachshund's ability to sleep in different positions.
- If your dachshund lies down for a nap, take the cart off.

Outside

- When she is in the cart, keep your dog on a leash if you are not in an enclosed area. She can get away from you very quickly!
- Attach the leash to the dog, not to the cart.
- Make sure the back feet do not drag.

wheelchair fun

That's right—fun! When you got your dog a wheelchair, you became part of a very elite club.

Races!

Your cart dog can compete in wheelchair races. Is there anything more adorable than a bunch of wiener dogs racing each other in their carts? I think not. See your local dachshund rescue website to see if they put on a race near you. (Pro tip: Practice your starts and finishes! Dachshund races are won by focus, not speed.)

Costumes!

If you're the sort of person who dresses your dog up at Halloween, imagine the new possibilities open to you. You can incorporate the wheelchair into the costume. I've seen wheelchairs dressed up as police cars, train engines, Snoopy's dog house, a pirate ship, and Santa's sleigh. Our dear friend Skippy used to go all over the country dressed as a John Deere tractor (mom Angela is the farmer) and a hotdog stand. Get those creative juices flowing (and send us your pictures).

Public Adoration!

It's great fun to take your wheelchair dog out for walks in public, especially in parks or at a street festival or fair. People go crazy for a dog in a wheelie cart, and your dachshund will likely bask in all the attention. Be ready to talk to people about your experience—they will want to talk to you! Here's your chance to be an ambassador for handicapped dogs everywhere.

sling, batter batter! an alternative to wheelchair carts

From the Desk of Dr. Christman

My Cosmo does not like using a cart. I have tried multiple types, but he seems to feel they are too heavy. However, he loves when we go on walks together with the sling I made for him out of a regular resistance band. The sling gives him the freedom to go wherever he wants, as fast as he wants, and I even get some great exercise keeping up with him.

These resistance bands are commercially available at any big box retailer. I simply put some bandaging material at the bottom of the loop so it doesn't rub his skin. The elasticity provides him the movement he needs. I just lift his rear legs off the ground a couple of inches so his rear feet do not drag.

If you cannot afford a cart, or if your small dog cannot use a cart for another reason, the resistance band may be a great alternative. Even my parents love walking Cosmo with it.

—Adam Christman, DVM, MBA

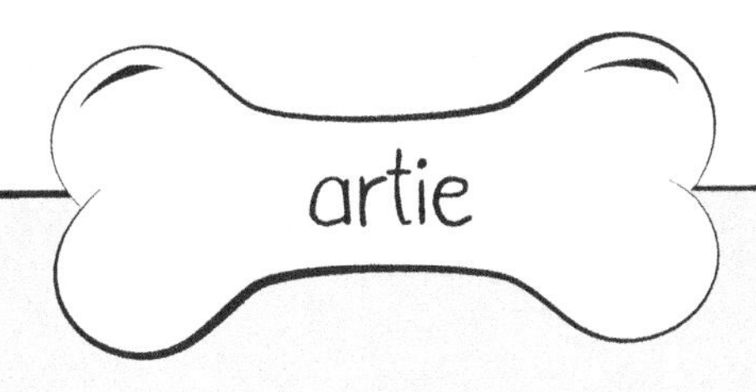

Artie the Wonder Dog

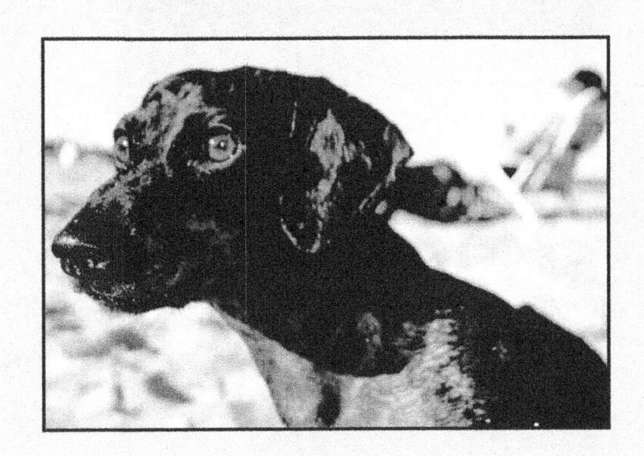

Artie's inability to use his back legs has never slowed him down. He still manages to keep up with our other dogs and any fosters who come and go.

Artie never meets a stranger, and his favorite adventures are at the off-leash beach in Boca Raton, Florida. On our first visit there, it was sensory overload when we first arrived. But then he got down in the sand and introduced himself to several new friends (dogs and people). Artie wasn't a big fan of the water, even though I made him test it out a few times, but he played, he swam, and he rested.

He is a fan of Home Depot (where Mommy works) and enjoys the sights and smells of lumber, kitchen and bath accessories, and power tools. Needless to say, he is a local Home Depot store favorite, where Mommy's friend Alvin adjusts his cart whenever he needs a "tune-up."

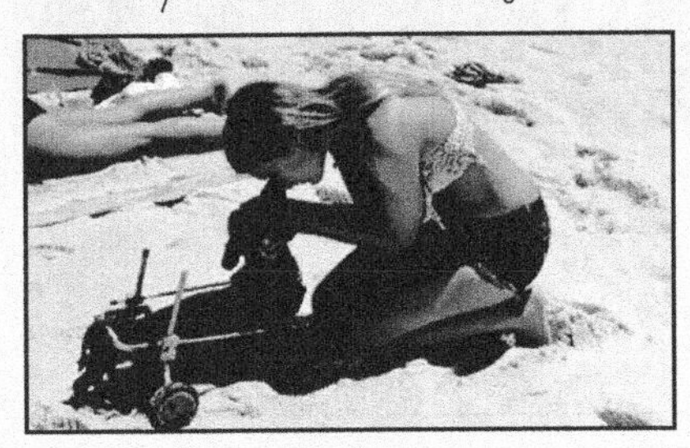

Artie is also our resident shoe thief. We have to make sure that all of our shoes are put away when we leave the room, because they are not safe otherwise. Sandals are his favorite chew toy.

Artie is roughly seven years old. We adopted him from the shelter shortly after he became paralyzed at age three.

—Rhonda Kaleta (Holly Springs, Georgia)

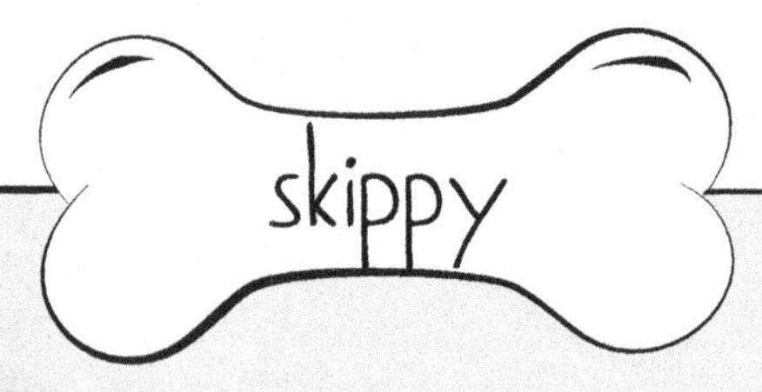

skippy

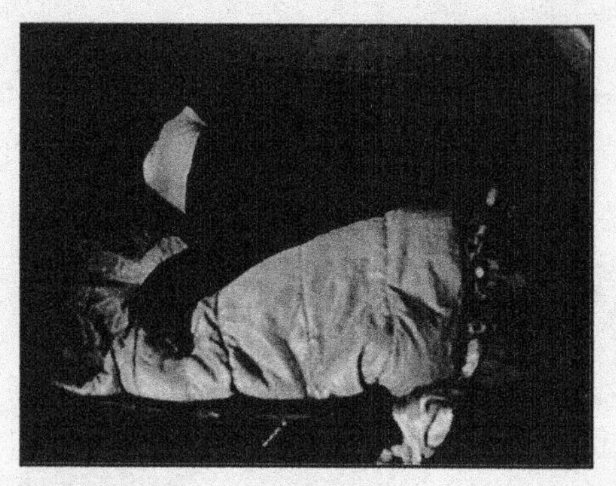

Skippy loved kids, and he especially loved how much attention kids gave him whenever he was out and about in his wheelie cart. One weekend, my niece and nephew were spending the night with me, and they wanted to pitch the tent in the guest room to sleep in. Skippy and I went to bed in my bedroom as usual, but when I got up in the middle of the night, I noticed Skippy was not in his bed. I found that he had sneaked out of our room and nosed open two doors to get to the kids so he could climb into the tent and "camp out" too, all snuggled up in the middle!

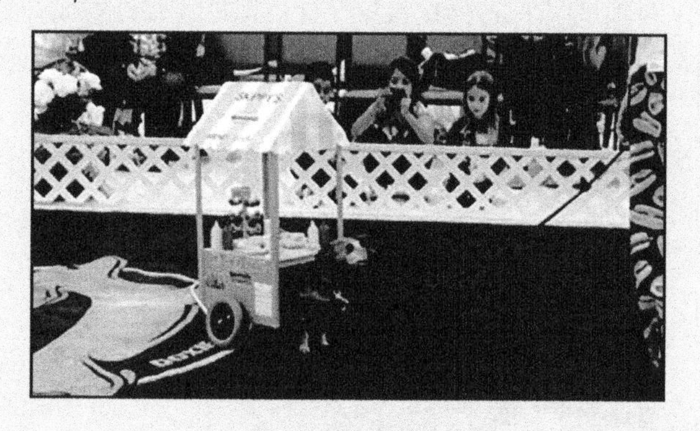

Skippy was also a racing champion, winning the National Dachshund Races five times from 2010 to 2015 (as well as the qualifying races to get there!). He died at age 14 after 12 years in his wheelie cart (and many handcrafted, lightweight wheelie cart costumes, including a John Deere tractor and a Varsity hot dog stand). After Skippy's death, I adopted another paralyzed dog, Maggie, who is also showing talent for wheelchair racing!

—Angela Johnston (Eufala, Alabama)

preparation tools, glossary, and other resources

preparation tools: minimizing your risk and being prepared

10 Ways to Minimize the Risk of an IVDD Event

You can't minimize the risk of IVDD itself. If your dachshund inherited the condition, she has it. You can, however, minimize the risk of the disease actually injuring the spinal cord.

1. No jumping. The most common event that pushes IVDD into a rupture is an impact. Don't allow your dachshund to jump off anything—including the couch and bed. Use a ramp so she can get off furniture by herself. Train her never to jump down without you.
2. No stairs—especially not down stairs. Every stair is a little jump. Every jump is a little impact to the back. Train your dachshund to wait for you at the top so you can carry her down. Block the stairs with a baby gate if you can't do the training.
3. Use a harness instead of a collar when you go on walkies (especially helpful if your dachshund is a puller). Harnesses distribute pressure more evenly, minimizing pressure on the cervical discs.
4. Support the back whenever you pick up your dachshund. Ask anyone who picks up your dachshund to use both hands and to support your dog's front and rear legs.
5. Support the back whenever you carry your dachshund. Use the "football" carry, with the dachshund's belly resting on the forearm and her butt tucked under your arm.
6. Keep nails trimmed. Long nails can make it easy to slip, and slips can trigger injuries.
7. Keep foot hair trimmed for long-haired dachshunds to minimize risk of slipping.
8. Maintain a healthy weight. Keep your dachshund on the skinny side, with a nice tuck at the waist. It is unclear whether obesity contributes to disc ruptures, but a dog with a rupture will have a much easier time recovering if she does not have to lift extra pounds with weak rear legs.
9. Investigate supplements for healthy cartilage and joints, but don't go supplement-crazy. Ask your veterinarian for recommendations. Some supplements should not be taken together, and others should not be taken by dogs with certain liver or kidney problems. Be smart.
10. Good nutrition, of course, is the basis for preventing many health problems, and IVDD is no exception. Keep your dog on a balanced diet with appropriate nutrients to encourage healthy cartilage and bones.

Nine Ways to Proactively Prepare for an IVDD Injury

1. Develop a relationship with a general practitioner veterinarian. You want to feel confident that your veterinarian knows your dachshund and you.
2. Have a proactive conversation about IVDD and dachshunds, and the vet's experience with them. Use the suggested questions on page 123 as a guide. Add other questions as you need to. Talk about this book and any concerns you thought of while reading it. Tell your veterinarian that you will be formulating an IVDD plan and that you want to talk to them about it when it is ready.
3. If you aren't comfortable with the conversation, for any reason, find another veterinarian. You want a good, dialogue-based relationship already in place with someone you trust *before* you need to make tough calls. Ask other dachshund owners, especially ones with IVDD experience, for veterinarian references.
4. Call the surgeons and emergency contacts on your vet's referral list to ask them for a general idea of pricing. Also find out whether they are available only by referral (during regular hours) or also for emergencies. Use the suggested questions on page 124 as a guide.
5. Create an IVDD plan using the templates starting on page 125. Discuss with your family as appropriate.
6. Discuss your IVDD plan with your regular vet, as well as your concerns and ideas about how you would probably want to handle different IVDD situations.
7. Crate train your dog. If she is already used to spending time in the crate, crate rest will be much less stressful for both of you, if she ever needs it.
8. Assemble your crate rest kit—even if you think you would opt for surgery. Your dog may have minor IVDD flare-ups that don't warrant surgery.
9. Memorize the signs of back pain. Make sure your family knows them too, and that they know to put your dachshund in the crate immediately if they see these signs.

Be proactive so that you do not have to be reactive.

Nine Key Signs of an IVDD Back Problem

Memorize these signs so that you can recognize potential IVDD as quickly as possible. Teach your family to recognize them too. If you suspect IVDD, put your dog in the crate immediately.

1. Yelping or crying
2. Trembling
3. Holding tummy muscles tight
4. Walking gingerly with a hunched back
5. Not getting out of bed in the morning (unless that is normal for your dachshund), not coming to greet you when you get home from work, or otherwise refusing to move
6. Refusing to go up or down stairs
7. Refusing to turn her head
8. Crying, squealing, flinching (or even snapping) when you touch her or pick her up
9. Can't support weight with back legs (obvious, I know)

Holding a "Let's Talk About IVDD" Conversation with Your Regular Veterinarian

There are no right or wrong answers to these questions, but a veterinarian's answers will give you a good feel for whether or not they are the right match for you. Most general practitioners will be happy to answer your questions during a regular office visit, but if you want to make a special appointment for the questions, you may have to pay for an office visit.

Introduction: "I'd like to be proactive and think through some of the possible IVDD scenarios so that I can make sure I am as prepared as possible in case anything happens."

Questions

1. What are some of your main observations about IVDD in dachshunds?
2. What advice about IVDD do you have for me as a dachshund owner?
3. What would happen if I brought my dog in and you thought it was IVDD? Would you refer me to a specialist, or would you recommend some other course of action?
4. What is your general philosophy on treating IVDD if the dog is not paralyzed? What if the dog is paralyzed?
5. How do you feel about conservative treatment or medical management of IVDD—strict crate rest with medications?
6. I'd like to call a couple of surgeons and find out more about them, so I have some options if I ever need to consider surgery. Where do you refer patients for IVDD surgery? Why do you like them?
7. When do you refer a neurologist instead of a surgeon?
8. What should I do if I think my dog is having back pain at a time when your office is closed?
9. What should I do if my dog becomes paralyzed at a time when your office is closed?

Holding a "Let's Talk about IVDD" Conversation with Potential Specialists

If you decide to consult with surgeons or neurologists in advance, you will probably need to make an appointment and pay for a professional consult.

Introduction: "I have a dachshund, and I'm very concerned about IVDD. I'd like to be proactive and think through some of the possible scenarios before anything happens, so I'm doing advance research into possible treatment options if an IVDD rupture happens to my dog. I got your contact information from my regular vet, Dr. ______________________, and I'd like to talk to you about IVDD."

Questions

1. What are some of your main observations about IVDD in dachshunds?
2. What advice about IVDD do you have for me as a dachshund owner?
3. Is IVDD surgery a common procedure in your practice?
4. What is your philosophy on surgery for dogs who are not paralyzed but have IVDD pain?
5. Do you prefer that the referring veterinarian use steroids or NSAIDs before a dog comes to you for IVDD surgery? Why is that your preference?
6. Does your practice take emergency surgeries, only scheduled referrals, or something else?
7. What could I expect to pay for diagnostics, a hemilaminectomy, and hospitalization for a typical dachshund at your practice, assuming no complications?
8. When do you recommend using a neurologist rather than your services?

IVDD plan worksheets

Electronic copies of the following worksheets are available on our website:

- My IVDD Plan: Regular Business Hours
- My IVDD Plan: Off Hours
- My IVDD Plan: Crate Rest Medications

After you have completed these worksheets, print all three sheets for your refrigerator. Keep a digital copy on your computer desktop, and give a copy to your veterinarian and your pet sitters. Make sure your family knows what to do in case something happens and you are not there to make the decisions.

MY IVDD PLAN: REGULAR BUSINESS HOURS

Name of Dog: ____

If I see signs of back pain during normal office hours, my plan is to...	
☐ Go to my regular vet to get meds for conservative crate rest treatment. ☐ Start conservative crate rest treatment. I already have the meds, and I know the doses and timing. ☐ Something else: ______________________	Name of Vet: Address: Phone Number: Hours:
If my dog becomes paralyzed during normal office hours, my plan is to...	
☐ Go to my regular vet to decide whether surgery or crate rest is the best option. ☐ Go to my regular vet to get the meds for conservative crate rest treatment. ☐ Start conservative crate rest with the meds I already have. ☐ Something else: ______________________	Name of Vet: Address: Phone Number: Hours:
If I decide to move forward with surgery during regular business hours, I want to be referred to...	
Name of Surgeon:	Address:
Phone Number:	Hours:
Other notes	
I talked to Dr. ________________ about how they handle surgeries. If you have a choice of anti-inflammatory medications, I'd prefer to use a steroid/NSAID **(circle one)** because Dr. ________________ told me that it ________________ ____	

MY IVDD PLAN: OFF HOURS

Name of Dog: ______________________________

If I see signs of back pain and my regular vet is closed, my plan is to...	
☐ Keep my dog in the crate until we can get to my regular vet tomorrow. Manage pain by ____________ ____________ ☐ Go to the emergency vet to get meds for conservative crate rest treatment. ☐ Start conservative crate rest treatment. I already have the meds. ☐ Something else: ____________	Name of Regular Vet: Address: Phone Number: Hours: Name of Emergency Vet: Address: Phone Number: Hours:

If my dog becomes paralyzed and my regular vet is closed, my plan is to...	
☐ Keep her in the crate until we can get to my vet tomorrow. Manage pain by ____________ ____________ ☐ Go to the emergency vet to decide whether surgery or crate rest is the best option. ☐ Start conservative crate rest treatment. I already have the meds. ☐ Something else: ____________	Name of Regular Vet: Address: Phone Number: Hours: Name of Emergency Vet: Address: Phone Number: Hours:

If I decide to move forward with surgery during emergency hours, I want to be referred to...	
Name of Surgeon:	Address:
Phone Number:	Hours:

Other notes
I talked to Dr. ____________ about how they handle surgeries. If you have a choice of anti-inflammatory medications, I'd prefer to use a steroid/NSAID **(circle one)** because Dr. ____________ told me that it ____________
If something happens on a Friday night (as opposed to a Sunday night), my answers are a little different: ____________ ____________
Instructions for my pet sitter if you cannot reach me: ____________

MY IVDD PLAN: CRATE REST MEDICATIONS

Your veterinarian may have reasons for not selecting a drug for your dog on any row. If you are concerned, try phrasing your question like this: "Is there a reason not to give a <type of drug>? If not, I would like to."

Type	Why Needed	Common Examples	What Did Your Vet Prescribe?
Anti-inflammatory (either steroidal or NSAID, but not both)	Reduce swelling and pressure on the spinal cord. Relieve pain.	Steroidal: • Prednisone • Dexamethasone • Prednisolone Non-steroidal (NSAID): • Deramaxx/deracoxib • Metacam/meloxicam • Previcox/firocoxib • Rimadyl/carprofen	Drug: Dose/Frequency: For how long?
Breakthrough pain medication	Relieve pain between anti-inflammatory doses. Note: May also have sedating effects. Some vets prescribe more than one.	• Ultram/tramadol • Amantadine • Neurontin/gabapentin	Drug: Dose/Frequency: For how long?
Muscle relaxant	Relax other muscles compensating for the back pain by tightening up–resulting in painful spasms. Note: May also have sedating effects.	• Robaxin/ methocarbamol • Diazepam	Drug: Dose/Frequency: For how long?
Sedative	Calm agitated dog so that she does not move around in the crate and prevent healing.	• Alprazolam • Acepromazine	Drug: Dose/Frequency: For how long?
Tummy soother	Prednisone and NSAIDs can cause gastrointestinal distress and bleeding. Stress can also cause tummy issues. A tummy soother is recommended from the beginning to prevent it. Some vets will advise that you use two.	• Pepcid AC (OTC)/ famotidine • Sucralfate	Drug: Dose/Frequency: For how long?

Back-up Plan: What should I do if my dog is in pain and your office is closed? ______________________________

For your pet sitter or family, if you are away:

Where are these medications stored? ______________________________

glossary: the language of IVDD

These informal definitions are by no means comprehensive, but they will help you understand what your veterinarian is saying and how to talk about your dog's IVDD with a bit more confidence. Some of these terms are not used in this book, but your veterinarian may use them.

Annulus fibrosus: The tough exterior coating of the intervertebral disc. This coating surrounds the jelly-like inner material. The annulus fibrosus in a dog with IVDD will be weaker and more brittle than in a normal dog.

Bulging disc: A disc that is swelling but has not actually broken through the fibrous coating.

C1 – C7: The discs in the neck (C stands for cervical). If your veterinarian says the problem is at C3, for example, that means the third disc in the neck.

Calcification: When the coating of a disc starts to get brittle. Some calcifications can actually show up on an x-ray. However, it's important to remember that the disc showing calcification may not be the disc actually causing the problem. Also known as *mineralization.*

Cervical region: The neck area. The seven discs in this region are labeled with a C. Note: Dogs with cervical disc problems will often cry out in pain when their heads are patted as a first sign of distress.

Chondrodystrophic: Dog breeds that have been selectively bred for a type of hereditary dwarfism that also creates a disorder of cartilage formation (and IVDD). Characteristics include angular limb deformities and abnormally short legs. Dachshunds are a classic example of a chondrodystrophic breed.

Compression: Disc bulge or rupture can behave in two ways as it harms the spinal cord. If the disc is simply pressing on the spinal cord, your vet may use the word compression. (Otherwise, your veterinarian may say percussion or concussion.)

Concussion: Sometimes called percussion. Disc rupture can behave in two ways as it harms the spinal cord. A concussion injury hits the spinal cord with more force than a compression injury does.

Conservative treatment: Crate rest with medications. Sometimes called medical management.

Computed Tomography (CT) scan: A diagnostic tool the veterinarian uses to pinpoint the specific discs affected in preparation for surgery. The CT scan produces one image from many x-ray images. The amount of gray in the image identifies tissues that are normal and abnormal. Some can produce a 3D image. Sometimes a dye is injected to increase the contrast. CT scans also can produce an image without the bone, as it can look at one "slice" of the body at a time.

Deep pain sensation (DPS): A dog's ability to perceive painful stimuli (for our purposes, in the rear feet). Vets will usually test for DPS by pinching the toes with a metal clamp. The ideal response is for the dog to pull back the foot and show recognition of the pain by crying or looking at the foot. Sometimes called deep pain perception (DPP).

Disc: The cushions in the space between the bones of the spine. Discs are composed of an outer fibrous coating called the annulus fibrosus and a gelatinous center called the nucleus pulposus.

Dura: The outer protective layer of the spinal cord. The dura has two purposes: protecting the delicate inner parts of the cord, and, through its many pain nerve fibers, letting the brain know something is wrong. Also known as the dura mater.

Explosive disc: A disc rupture that sends a small plug of disc material into the spinal cord at a high velocity (like a bullet), causing a percussion injury. Equivalent to Hansen Type III and traumatic IVDD.

Extrusion: When the jelly-like material inside the disc actually spurts out of a weak point in the disc coating. Same as herniation and a ruptured disc.

Fenestration: When the surgeon cuts a window in the vertebra to relieve pressure on the inflamed spinal cord, as part of a hemilaminectomy procedure. (Remember your high school Latin? *Fenestra* means window.)

Hansen Type I: The type of IVDD common in small and chondrodystrophic dogs. Dogs with Hansen Type I commonly first show signs when they are young to middle-aged, although signs can appear at any age.

Hansen Type III: A term some vets use to refer to a disc rupture that sends a small plug of disc material into the spinal cord at a high velocity (like a bullet). Equivalent to explosive disc and traumatic IVDD. It is actually a variation of Hansen Type I. (Yes, there is a Hansen Type II, but it is not related to IVDD.)

Hemilaminectomy: The most common surgical procedure to relieve pressure on the spinal cord from a disc rupture in the thoracic region. The surgeon uses a high-speed drill to remove a piece of vertebral bone. This allows the surgeon to see the spinal cord and remove any ruptured disc material. Creating the window (fenestration) and removing the disc material relieves the pressure on the spinal cord, allowing healing to start.

Herniation: When the jelly-like material inside the disc actually spurts out of a weak point in the disc coating. Same as extrusion and a ruptured disc.

L1 – L7: The discs in the lumbar region (just above the tail). If your veterinarian says the problem is at L7, for example, that means the lowest disc in this region.

Lesion: The spot where the disc is bulging or has ruptured.

Lumbar region: The region of the spine just above the tail. The seven discs in this region are labeled with an L.

Medical management: Crate rest with medications. Sometimes called conservative treatment.

Mineralization: Another term for calcification.

MRI: A diagnostic tool the veterinarian uses to pinpoint the specific discs affected in preparation for surgery. An MRI is the gold standard for diagnosing and pinpointing an IVDD disc. MRIs can image soft tissues and evaluate neural tissues. General anesthesia is required because the dog has to be absolutely still for 10 to 60 minutes. It's often available only at a referral hospital or a veterinary teaching hospital, and it's the most expensive of the diagnostics. An MRI is the only diagnostic tool reliably able to see edema (fluid buildup). This is important in understanding the prognosis for recovery.

Myelogram/myelography: A diagnostic tool the veterinarian uses to pinpoint the specific discs affected in preparation for surgery. General anesthesia is required. The veterinarian injects dye into the spinal cord and discs so that they will be visible on an x-ray. In some places, myelograms are more readily available and less expensive than an MRI or CT scan.

Myelomalacia (focal): Localized death of a specific spot in the spinal cord.

Myelomalacia (progressive): The progressive death of the spinal cord following a trauma (in this case, the compression or percussion from a disc). If myelomalacia is moving upward from the point of injury toward the head, it is called ascending. If it is moving downward, it is called descending.

Neurologic exam: A full neurologic exam includes many sections, giving the veterinarian a significant amount of information about whether and how to diagnose IVDD and how to recommend treatment. These tests also give the vet an approximation of which disc(s) in the back are affected.

Nucleus pulposus: The inner core of the disc, made up of a jelly-like material that acts as a cushion between the vertebrae. In a dog experiencing an IVDD, the nucleus pulposus will be bulging or ruptured, putting pressure on the spinal cord.

Paraplegia/paraplegic: Inability to walk with the rear legs.

Paresis: Weakness or partial loss of voluntary movement (in this case, in the rear legs).

Percussion: Sometimes called concussion. A percussion injury hits the spinal cord with more force than a compression injury does.

Polydipsia: Excessive or unusual thirst. Common in dogs who are taking prednisone, but can also be a symptom of an endocrine or metabolic condition unrelated to IVDD (e.g., diabetes, Cushing's disease, and kidney disease) especially common in dachshunds. Some IVDD dogs may concurrently have these conditions, so it is important to check with your veterinarian about unusual water intake.

Proprioception: A dog's ability to know where the feet are and to correct their placement.

Ruptured disc: When the jelly-like material inside the disc actually spurts out of a weak point in the disc coating. Same as herniation and extrusion.

Slipped disc: A common term for a ruptured disc.

Spinal walking: Reflexive step-like movements that sometimes occur in dogs without deep pain sensation. Also known as "back walking." In spinal walking, the dog cannot coordinate the front and rear leg movements with each other. Some dogs with spinal walking do learn to get around with these involuntary movements, but it should not be confused with the actual ability to walk.

Swollen disc: See bulging disc.

T1 – T13: The discs in the thoracic region (the middle of the back). If your veterinarian says the problem is at T4, for example, that means the fourth disc in this region.

Thoracic region: The region in the middle of your dog's back. Sometimes called the thoracolumbar region. The 13 discs in this region are labeled with a T.

Traumatic IVDD: A term some vets use to refer to a disc rupture that sends a small plug of disc material into the spinal cord (like a bullet) at a high velocity. Equivalent to explosive disc and Hansen Type III.

Urinary tract infection (UTI): Dogs with limited mobility are prone to infections of the bladder. An ascending UTI is one that is migrating upward from the bladder through the ureters to the kidneys.

Ventral slot: A surgical procedure often used for cervical discs. The surgeon approaches the disc from under the chin and creates an opening into the spinal column with a drill to relieve the pressure and remove any ruptured disc material.

X-rays/radiographs: Because discs and the spinal cord are not bone, x-rays are extremely limited tools for diagnosing IVDD. Vets often use x-rays to rule out other causes for a dog's symptoms. An x-ray can show two hints that support a diagnosis of IVDD: abnormal vertebrae spacing or calcification. Abnormal spacing indicates a disc rupture. Calcification supports a general diagnosis of IVDD the disease, although the disc showing calcification may not be the disc actually causing problems.

resources

Websites and Facebook Pages

- Our website (www.honeyhaveyousqueezedthedachshund.com) and Facebook page include electronic versions of the worksheets in this book, links to additional information sources, and listings of events relevant to IVDD.
- Dodgerslist (www.dodgerslist.com) has assembled a treasure trove of IVDD information over several years, with many people contributing their knowledge and personal experience. This website is quite comprehensive, containing IVDD information at many levels of detail and medical sophistication. It includes links to the latest research studies as well as recommended surgeons and veterinary teaching hospitals. Dodgerslist manages a Facebook page and an active online community support forum (see below). *Bottom line: If you have an IVDD dog, you need to be on Dodgerslist.*
- K9BackPack (www.k9backpack.com) provides a wealth of information about IVDD. It is the labor of love of a small group of friends who met online by sharing their stories about their dachshunds with IVDD. K9BackPack also manages a Facebook community page.
- The Veterinary Information Network's VeterinaryPartner.com site (www.veterinarypartner.com) allows you to email questions to their veterinarians and other specialists.

Supportive Communities

You will feel much better when you realize you and your dog are not facing IVDD alone. Several online communities hold ongoing conversations about their challenges with IVDD. They would love to hear your stories and share their experiences with you.

- The Dodgerslist Care and Support Forum (http://dodgerslist.boards.net) responds very quickly to questions and concerns from members. Once you are a member, you will receive quick, knowledgeable, and supportive responses to your questions about IVDD—and no question is too small or too large for them to handle graciously. The volunteer moderators, while not veterinarians, have extensive knowledge and hands-on experience. You will also receive input from other forum members. Different perspectives will help you to make smart decisions for your dog.
- Facebook groups: The Facebook group that focuses specifically on discussions of IVDD is called IVDD and Other Back Disorders. You will find a supportive (and opinionated!) community of people eager to commiserate with you. Facebook has several other groups dedicated to those who love dachshunds in general. On all of these groups, people discuss dachshund back problems (as well as share a lot of pictures of their adorable dogs and funny stories about their adventures). Some examples are Dachshund Lovers, Doxie Posse, and Dachshunds Rock! New groups seem to pop up regularly.
- Twitter: Use the hashtag #IVDD to find people talking about their dogs' back issues and life with an IVDD dog—very often a dachshund, of course. Follow the @K9BackPack Twitter handle for lots of IVDD information. The K9BackPack folks are quick to respond to Twitter questions. Dodgerslist also runs a Twitter account (@DodgersList). You can follow us at @HHYSTD and @NJ_Chico.

Wheelchair Cart Sources

- Dewey's Wheelchairs for Dogs (www.wheelchairsfordogs.com)
- Doggon' Wheels (www.doggonwheels.com)
- Eddie's Wheels (www.eddieswheels.com)
- K9 Carts (www.k9carts.com)
- Ruff Rollin' (www.ruffrollin.com)
- Walkin' Wheels (www.walkinwheels.com) has several resellers. Our favorite is www.handicappedpets.com.
- Best Friend Mobility (www.bestfriendmobility.org)
- Dogs To Go (www.dogstogo.net)
- The Rolling Dog Project (Facebook)

Crate Training

It is never too late to crate train. A crate-trained dog will have a much easier time adjusting to crate rest if she doesn't have to simultaneously get used to being crated for the first time. Use only positive methods! These site have terrific tips on crate training adult dogs:

- www.dodgerslist.com (includes emergency version for the IVDD dog not previously crate trained)
- www.whole-dog-journal.com
- www.positively.com
- www.dehumane.org
- www.cesarsway.com
- www.atlantahumane.org

Financing Surgery

If finances are a barrier, talk to your surgeon about ways to keep costs as low as possible without compromising care or pain management. Most people who cannot directly fund their dog's surgery use a combination of the below methods.

1. Borrowing
    - CareCredit payment plan
    - Friends and family
2. Online fundraising: Online fundraisers need great photos. Use a photo of your dog from before her injury and one of her in the hospital. Do frequent updates with more photos. Publicize it on Facebook.
    - gofundme.com
    - youcaring.com
3. Personal fundraising: People seem to respond very well to fundraising campaigns in which the person asking for funds is making an effort (like holding an event or making homemade goods) and not just asking for a donation. Many supporters will make an additional contribution in these cases.
    - Hold a fundraising event (chili cook-off, yard sale, bake sale)
    - Sell homemade goods to friends (soaps, pastas, jellies, sauces)

closing thoughts

will IVDD be around forever?

We humans created IVDD as we selectively bred dogs for cute dwarf characteristics to develop specific breeds like dachshunds. That cuteness brought along some unexpected ugly baggage for the ride—namely, faulty cartilage and discs.

With some careful thought and commitment, I believe that we can drastically reduce the prevalence of IVDD in the breeds we love.

> IVDD is congenital. We humans control the breeding.

You can do three things to move the needle on IVDD in that direction. The first two involve making some noise. The last one involves contributing to the body of knowledge for researchers working on this disease.

1. Notify your breeder. If you purchased your dachshund at a breeder, tell them that they have IVDD in their gene pool. Request that they stop breeding that mother and father. Request it in writing and with a phone call.

   Expect a variety of reactions to your request. Some will dismiss your concerns as unavoidable or unpredictable. Some will say that IVDD just isn't trackable in that way. Some will say that it isn't that simple. Some will say taking those dachshunds out of the gene pool would just shrink the pool further and create other problems. Some may say that they just can't worry about that.

   Some of these reactions have a level of validity, but we need to start somewhere—and I believe that the starting point is to not breed dogs that we know have this propensity. There is certainly no shortage of dachshunds for the breeding pool now. You will learn a lot about your breeder from their response.

2. Notify the registering organization. Squeak, squeak, squeak that wheel! Report your dachshund's IVDD to the American Kennel Club (AKC), Canadian Kennel Club (CKC), or whoever issued your dog's registration papers. Ask that they stop registering puppies from those parents. CC them on the letter you sent to your breeder.

We know that IVDD is passed down. A breeder who truly cares about the betterment of the breed, and the puppies they create, would take any precautions needed to make sure they are not pushing more IVDD genes out into the world to reproduce. Any pedigree organization with a mission statement that includes the words "advance canine health and well-being," "health and welfare," or "protecting and promoting the health and welfare" should be on top of this.

If enough of us complain, they may do something about it. As long as we are quiet, registering organizations have no reason to change anything. They receive their revenue from registration fees.

3. Participate in research projects. Vet schools conduct ongoing IVDD studies that require data about dogs with the disease. You can add your dachshund's genetic information (through a blood or saliva sample) to that body of knowledge or answer survey questions.

IVDD and further advances in treatment

From the Desk of Dr. Christman

Even we veterinarians ask ourselves, "Does this dog need surgical or medical intervention?" every day when we see a dog with back issues. Intervertebral disc disease should, ideally, be considered a surgical disease. However, it would be naive to consider all cases as necessarily surgical cases. The question is rather one of if the spinal cord were compressed, would it not be ideal to decompress it before further or permanent damage occurs? Medical therapy is directed at reducing spinal cord swelling, providing pain relief, and attempting to prevent further protrusion or extrusion of disc material by restricting activity (that is, crate rest). The hope is that confinement allows for tears in the annulus fibrosus to heal, and that the extruded disc material is soft enough to spread around the spinal cord and no longer act as a compressive mass. Many "long back" dogs, such as dachshunds, with cervical disc extrusions exhibit only pain, despite considerable compression of the cervical spine. In contrast, even small compressions of the T3–L3 cord will result in neurological deficits. Delaying decompression often results in adhesions to the dura, making later removal more challenging and potentially less successful in restoring function. Successful medical management is also often temporary, and most reports indicate that at least 30 to 50 percent return with a recurrence of signs and therapeutic failure.

Considering the length of the canine spine, and the natural thoracolumbar fulcrum, compared to humans where the spinal cord ends at L1–L2, paralysis from disc extrusion is more likely in dogs and warrants early surgical intervention. Contact your breeder to notify them that this issue has happened. Breeding professionals should be striving every day to provide healthy genetic lines for the future.

As of this writing, many research studies are currently working with stem cell therapies. Ask your local veterinarian about them. Iowa State University's and North Carolina State University's Colleges of Veterinary Medicine are performing clinical trials enlisting dogs with IVDD. Stem cells have the ability to rapidly multiply and to take on the functions of specialized cells by assimilation. A sample of adipose (fat) tissue and sensory nerves are taken from the back of a dog's neck, from which stem cells and particular nerve cells (called Schwann cells) are cultured. The therapy involves injecting the combination of stem cells and Schwann cells directly into the injured area in the spine. Results have been fascinating. This could soon be a viable alternative to surgery.

—Adam Christman, DVM, MBA

you're an ambassador now

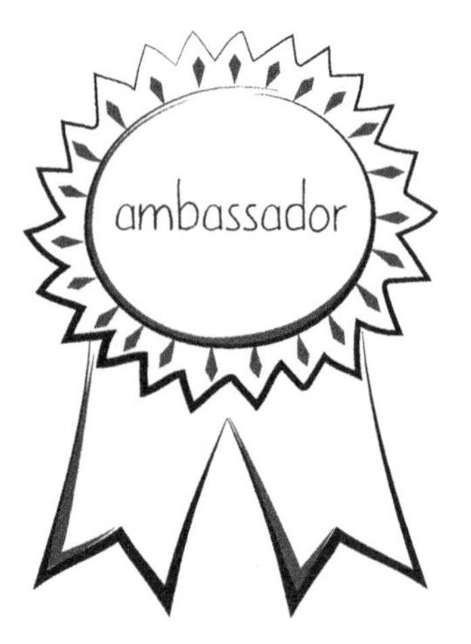

Your attitude toward your dog can save other dogs' lives. Most people are not used to seeing disabled dogs—in fact, many people have never seen one.

This is one of the things society seems to hide from itself very well.

You can save more dachshund lives by making your happy disabled dachshund (and your happy attitude about it) visible. You never know when someone whose dog has just gone down will remember that they saw you and realize that maybe there is hope for their dog, or their friend's dog, or their brother's dog.

Take your IVDD dachshund out into the world. Let people see her—her joy, her adaptability, her quality of life. Answer their questions with an open, honest, glad face. If they ask, be matter-of-fact about the special care required.

When people say, "Oh, how sad!" tell them, "She's not sad at all! She's just a dog doing her dog thing. She doesn't even seem to remember that she's any different from before."

If your dachshund walks, get a T-shirt for her that says "I recovered from IVDD. Ask me about it."

If your dachshund drags, take her to dog parks and grassy areas to play, and get ready for the questions! Let people see her thumping around the grass to follow you or chase a ball. Let them see how happy both of you are.

Most people will think that a dog in a wheelchair is cute. A dog dragging along the grass, on the other hand, is not what people expect to see. Prepare yourself for some different reactions. This will be the first time most people have seen a dog like this, and they may not always be tactful. This is your chance to practice kindness and show people that dogs with disabilities do exist and are content.

And although you are an ambassador, remember that other people's attitudes are not your responsibility. I once had a man tell me that my dachshund (who was chasing a ball and barking her head off with joy at the time) was "suffering." I knew I wasn't going to change his mind. So I just said, "She seems happy playing, doesn't she?" and left it at that.

You may be able to plant only a seed. But some seeds grow great things.

dogs and people to thank

For all the IVDD dogs I have loved, fostered, and coached—online, by phone, and in the real world. You gave me so much joy—both in caring for you, and in puzzling out how to make that care better and easier for all of us. Most especially, Tabby, Jack, and Paris, who shared my life and my home as "permanent staff."

To the DREAM Dachshund Rescue board members and foster homes, past and present, who have saved so many dachshund lives through their compassionate hearts for dogs and people.

To the wonderful folks at Dodgerslist, K9BackPack, and the IVDD and Other Back Disorders Facebook group. You have saved more lives than you will ever be able to count. Special thanks to Linda Stowe, Paula Milner, and Regina Reif for their detailed reviews and wise counsel.

To my writing group, Craig Bryant, Wendy Kinney, Lara Lowman, Nicki Salcedo, Jill Pullen, and Michelle Newcome, for their unending encouragement and wise counsel. Thank you for never hinting, not even through a raised eyebrow, that a book about disabled dachshunds was far too specific to be worth anyone's while. And for patiently providing your feedback at a table surrounded by paraplegic dachshunds begging for attention.

Two teachers stand out: My 7th and 8th grade English teacher, Mrs. Bragdon, who taught me to love language and its rules, and Dr. Ray Wallace, my first technical writing professor at the University of Tennessee. His paper airplanes flew in a direct line to the IVDD dachshund bladders.

To Dr. Christman, for his openness to collaborating on this book. When I first saw his love and can-do attitude for Cosmo on his social media channels, I cheered out loud. I knew he was the perfect veterinary writing partner. I am so grateful he was willing to take a chance on the crazy lady from Twitter and read my initial chapters with care and good spirit.

Most of all, to Craig, for telling me that this book is important, that I needed to write it, and not letting me quit. For learning with me, and never failing to make me laugh about things most people would cry about.

—Kristin Leydig Bryant

I have been inspired by IVDD dogs ever since I was in veterinary school. Their strength, their fortitude, and their willing need to see life the same way as any other dog sees it never cease to amaze and inspire me. These dogs are the reason I continue to do what I love every day.

To all my patients and non-patients (blogs, social media, rescue organizations), thank you for making me a better person and a compassionate veterinarian. Being a veterinarian is one of the most difficult careers on this Earth—emotions run high, death happens overwhelmingly, finances have bearing on outcomes, the value of a pet is deemed differently in each individual's eyes, and so much more. But one thing is certain—we all love and cherish our furbabies.

I want to personally thank my paralyzed dachshund/son, Cosmo, for giving me the inspiration to help the IVDD dogs out there and realize that life is just as beautiful even when you can't walk. Cosmo, you are my hero and will always be with me in my heart! To my other three furbabies, Charles, Chelsea, and Connor, you are the other three chambers to my heart. Thank you for being in my life and allowing me to mush you up and be both your daddy and your doctor. I love you all so much. You are my world.

To my fiancé, Chris: You have been with me through so many trials and tribulations in my career, and I could not have done it without your love and support. Our "children" love you so much, as much as I do. Thank you for everything!

And finally, to my family, and especially my parents: Mom and Dad, you have supported my journey of becoming a veterinarian since I was a child. Thank you for allowing your son to pursue his dream and passion. Not many can say that they found their passion in life, and I did because of the two of you. You are my best friends, my rock, and my everything. Thank you for being my number one fans! Thank you to my brother Tom and my nephews Gavin and Logan for continuing to share the love and passion of animals. I love you guys!

Thank you, Kristin Leydig Bryant, for having the courage and the dedication to put this book together. I would not have wanted to do this with anyone but you! Congratulations! We finally did it!

—Adam Christman, DVM, MBA

about the authors and illustrator

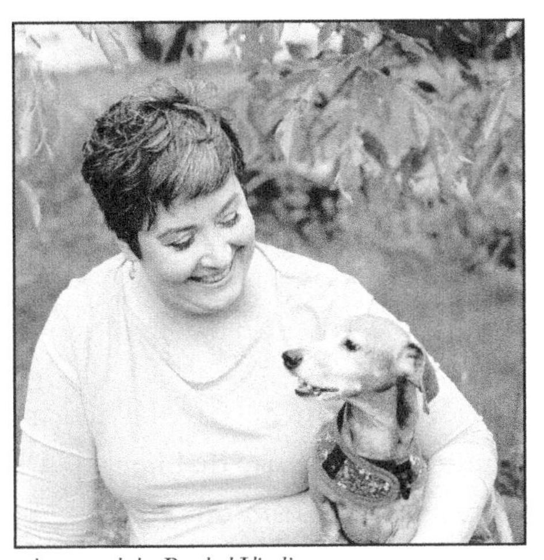

photograph by Rachel Iliadis

Kristin Leydig Bryant

Kristin began volunteering with dachshund rescue in 2002. Before that time, she had been intrigued by pictures of IVDD dachshunds in their wheelie carts and was curious about what it would take to care for a dog with disabilities.

In 2004, Kristin agreed to foster a "down" dachshund whose family could not provide medical care. She met the little dog's owners in the parking lot of an outlet mall, where they handed over a reeking bundle wrapped in pee pads and duct tape. The dog inside could barely lift her head, but she did make eye contact. The family told Kristin that eight days before, their vet had sent them home with prednisone and no other instructions. This meant that Tabby, as Kristin named her, had not emptied her bladder for eight days. The pee pads were soaked with stale overflow urine, feces, and blood from the intestinal ulcerations caused by the steroid.

Tabby and Kristin learned together, and Kristin found that she loved working with these dogs. Over the next few years, as she fostered other IVDD dogs (we stopped counting after seven), she became the "go-to" person at DREAM Dachshund Rescue who made surgery and crate rest decisions for IVDD foster dogs, took them to rehab, and coached people who contacted DREAM for help with their own dogs. In 2007, one of Kristin's other dachshunds, Jack, became paralyzed from IVDD. His surgery was unsuccessful, but he lived another six years and even hunted critters successfully in the backyard after his injury. Since then, Kristin has fostered many other dogs with IVDD and adopted a second paraplegic dachshund, Paris. Kristin has coached hundreds of people in person and virtually on caring for dachshunds with IVDD.

Kristin lives in Atlanta, Georgia, with her husband Craig. Their family experiences firsthand the full and joyous life possible for a paraplegic dachshund. Tabby lived to be 17 and loved to sleep tucked under Kristin's arm each night. Paris, now 10, likes to burrow to the bottom of the bed, sometimes falling off the end into the "hammock" made by the tucked-in sheet.

When she is not enjoying home life with her husband and dogs, Kristin works as a consultant specializing in organizational change management.

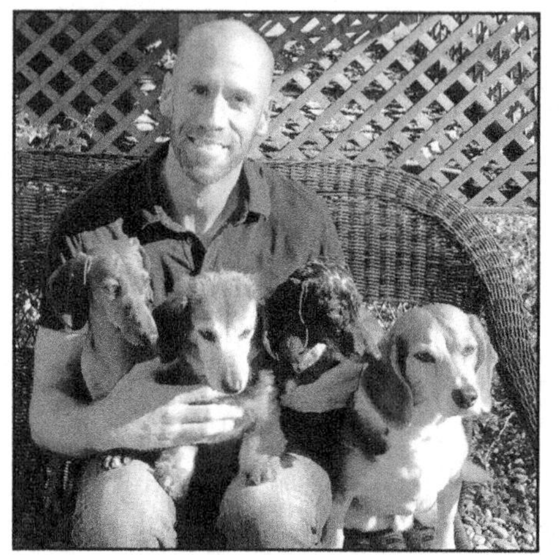

photograph by Christopher Zisko

Dr. Adam Christman, DVM, MBA

Dr. Christman has had a fond attachment to dogs with back problems beginning with his neurology rotation at Iowa State University College of Veterinary Medicine. After his rotation, he furthered his skills by taking rehabilitation classes to gain a greater sense of respect for these guys and their possibilities.

Upon completion of veterinary school, Dr. Christman started practicing in his home state of New Jersey. He anticipated the day that he would encounter another IVDD dog, and sure enough, Cosmo, a beautiful, red, long-haired dachshund, came in to his practice. Cosmo's owners were unable to afford his surgery and turned guardianship over to Dr. Christman. Although Cosmo had lost deep pain sensation before surgery, Dr. Christman, hopeful, moved forward with a hemilaminectomy. After months of rehabilitation, including acupuncture, underwater treadmill, and massage, however, Cosmo's paralysis was permanent.

Nine years later, Dr. Christman is still madly in love with Cosmo. He also has two other dachshunds and a beagle, who are his world. Recently, Dr. Christman was in the rehabilitation process with a dapple dachshund, Chelsea, who had L1, L2, L3 hemilaminectomy surgery. She is walking and doing beautifully!

Dr. Christman believes strongly in the human-animal bond and will do anything he can to strengthen that relationship. He loves helping dogs with special needs and disabilities, and he especially enjoys showcasing IVDD dogs, including Cosmo, on his YouTube channel to demonstrate how easy caring for these wonderful, loving creatures can be.

Dr. Christman has practiced veterinary medicine for more than 13 years and is Co-Chief of Staff at Brick Town Veterinary Hospital in Brick, New Jersey.

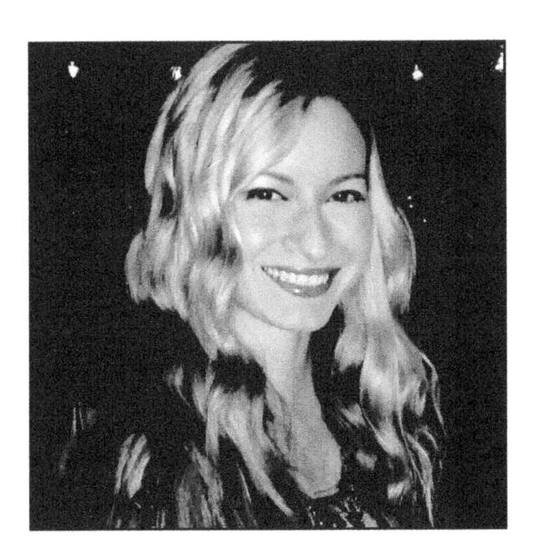

Kelly Guntner

Growing up in Paris, Texas, Kelly was a small-town girl with a big imagination. She knew from the moment she hung her first sketch on the fridge that she was destined to be an artist. Winning an art scholarship sealed her destiny. After graduating from Texas A&M University–Corpus Christi with a B.A. in Art and an emphasis in graphic design, she spent four years painting commissioned requests and freelancing as a graphic designer to perfect her skills.

Having family in both Texas and Georgia, Kelly always had a fondness for Atlanta. That certainly made the transition easier when she moved there in 2014 for a job opportunity. Things she loves about Atlanta: the art and music scene; the weather and outdoor activities like biking, hiking the trails, and climbing Stone Mountain; and the outdoor festivals (the Dogwood and Yellow Daisy are among her favorites). She also really appreciates how close the airport is (in Paris, the closest airport was two hours away).

Kelly splits her time between bringing visual communication to a new level for business documentation, and illustrating how-to books in a charming way that fully engages the reader in the subject. Her ability to notice small details and highlight them in her art lends itself to the personal creations she paints in her spare time.

Kelly resides in Decatur, Georgia and bikes often to the Decatur Square for festivals. She doesn't currently have a dog, but some day... some day.

sources consulted

https://www.acvs.org/small-animal/intervertebral-disc-disease

http://www.animalmedcenter.com/faqs/category/intervertebral-disc-disease

http://www.cvmbs.colostate.edu/vetneuro/Neuro_exam/neuroExam.html

http://www.dogfoodadvisor.com

http://www.ivis.org/proceedings/navc/2005/SAE/225.pdf?LA=1